The Essential Guide
– to the –
OSPE
Assessments

The Essential Guide - to the - OSPE Assessments

First Edition

Editors

Arian Arjomandi Rad
MBBS / BSc student
Imperial College London School of Medicine

Robert Vardanyan
MBBS / BSc student
Imperial College London School of Medicine

Authors

Arian Arjomandi Rad
MBBS / BSc student
Imperial College London School of Medicine
- Basic Life Support
- The Cardiovascular System
- The Basis of Medical Imaging

Robert Vardanyan
MBBS / BSc student
Imperial College London School of Medicine
- The Anatomy and Examinations of the Upper Limb
- The Anatomy and Examinations of the Lower Limb

Seungmin Han
MBBS / BSc student
Imperial College London School of Medicine
- The Respiratory System

Samuel Hammond
MBBS / BSc student
Imperial College London School of Medicine
- Head, Neck, and Spine

Junzheng Wang
MBBS / BSc student
Imperial College London School of Medicine
- Clinical Communication

Vasiliki Kalogianni
MBBS / BSc student
Imperial College London School of Medicine
- The Anatomy and Examination of the Abdomen

OPERATION MEDICAL SCHOOL
71-75 Shelton Street,
Covent Garden,
London,
WC2H 9JQ

The Essential Guide to the OSPE Assessments ISBN: 978-1-5272-3356-0

Design cover: Inga Vardanyan
Illustrations: Kenhub

Printed in the United Kingdom

Acknowledgments

We are honoured to have collaborated with and received support from our esteemed panel of accreditors and reviewers, who provided us with invaluable support in writing this book and ensuring accurate and high quality content. In particular, we would like to thank:

Professor Keyoumars Ashkan
Consultant Neurosurgeon
BA (Hons.), BSc (Hons.), Dip Mus, MB BCh (Commend.), MD, MRCP (UK), FRCS (Eng.), FRCP, FRCPS (Glasg.), FRCS (SN)

Professor Brian Gazzard
Consultant Gastroenterologist
CBE, MA, MD, FRCP

Professor Kenneth Macleod
Professor of Cardiac Physiology, Imperial College London

Dr Vahram Harutyunyan
Consultant in Acute and Geriatric Medicine
MBBS (Equiv), MRCP (UK)

Dr Jennifer Quint
Consultant Respiratory Physician
MSc, PhD, FHEA ,FRCP

Dr Emanuele Sartori Instructor
Director, Facilitator, and Instructor
Italian Resuscitation Council
European Resuscitation Council

The European Resuscitation Council

EUROPEAN RESUSCITATION COUNCIL

Dr Alessandro Trevisan
Director, Facilitator, Instructor, and Educator
Italian Resuscitation Council
European Resuscitation Council

The Italian Resuscitation Council

IRC

Dr Luigi Langella
Director, Facilitator, and Instructor
Italian Resuscitation Council
European Resuscitation Council

With thanks to Michal Kawka, our pre-clinical coordinator, in helping strategise this project.

With our utmost gratitude to Kenhub for allowing our project to take form seamlessly. Kenhub is an online anatomy teaching platform with video tutorials, quizzes, articles and an extensive atlas. We thank them for contributing their high quality illustrations to The Essential Guide to the OSPE Assessments.

KEN HUB

BMA

We would also like to thank the British Medical Association for their invaluable support with the production of our book. Were it not for the help of the BMA, this book would have been finished in triple the time.

We are further grateful to the Medical Defence Union for their crucial sponsorship of the book. Our initial progress stems from the marketing, advice, and monetary support that was given to us by the MDU.

MDU

Introduction

The Essential Guide to the OSPE Assessments is an Imperial College London student-generated scientific and clinical textbook which comprehensively guides pre-clinical medical students through their Objective Structured Practical Examinations (OSPE) and assists them further in their learning of the pre-clinical medical curriculum.

The OSPE assessments are some of the first clinical examinations that medical students undertake before proceeding onto their clinical years. Students have to apply their surface anatomy knowledge, clinical communication skills, and examination techniques on patients, and the assessment is designed to equip students with the confidence and knowledge to perform the same tasks in a hospital setting. This book is an in-depth guide to approaching these fundamental examinations.

Moreover, we hope to make the process for those transitioning into their clinical years smoother by discussing relevant clinical cases and good medical practice, alongside the key information required to score maximal marks at each station of the exam. Therefore, the lack of a comprehensive learning resource which would aid in guiding pre-clinical medical students through their journey from lecture based "pre-clinical years" to their clinical years was at the basis of our work.

The book has been directed around learning outcomes set by previous exam takers to illustrate to students what they should aim to achieve, and we will explore each learning outcome with the key medical and scientific knowledge and high quality anatomical diagrams and illustrations. Specifcally, this book will cover the relevant anatomy of the systems involved in the examinations, the clinical skills involved in examining the systems, the doctor-patient approach and clinical communication skills needed by medical students dealing with a patient, all accompanied by specific and relevant examples. Furthermore, the learning outcome will have sections of 'Good Medical Practice' and 'Extra Knowledge' which will provide the reader with knowledge about pathologies, clinical scenarios and advices on how to outstand in the OSPE.
The pathologies and clinical cases explored directly link to the essential knowledge required by the students. Indeed, we truly hope to encourage the readers of the book to apply this 'explorational' approach we offer throughout their learning in medical school and their careers as future health practitioners.

The topics which will be covered by the book will be Clinical Communication; Cardiovascular Sciences: Respiratory system; Abdominal system; Head, Neck and Spine; Upper and Lower Limbs; Basic Life Support. Additionally, a short over-view of Medical Imaging techniques and their applications in clinical setting will be covered, accompanied by examples and illustrations for each type of imaging modality covered.

As we have been striving to produce a learning resource of great educational value and high accuracy for students we had the honour to get our book accredited and reviewed by the a panel of experts in the field of clinical medicine. We would like to particularly thank the European Resuscitation Council (ERC) for having accredited and reviewed sections of our work.

Arian Arjomandi Rad & Robert Vardanyan

Contents

To Dr Hoshang Arjomandi Rad, Shirin Mohammadi, and Rastin

I would like to thank them for the constant support and motivation that they have always given me, and I would like to dedicate my efforts within this book to them.

- Arian Arjomandi Rad

I attribute all my work and dedication in making this book to the support of my considerate family - Armen, Bella, & Inga Vardanyan. Իմ գանձեր:

- Robert Vardanyan

The Basic Life Support Station

By Arian Arjomandi Rad

Introduction to the chapter

Unlike all other practical skills tested in the OSPE, basic life support (BLS) skills will be sufficient to save a life in certain acute settings. Mastering BLS skills will ensure that you are part of a coordinated system of response which will increase the chances of survival of patients with out-of-hospital cardiac arrest.

Although I would not go so far as to say the skills learnt for BLS are the most complex in understanding and practice, I must again stress that being confident and performing well in this station will not only be essential to pass the exam, but it will empower you to save lives. For this reason, it's sad to think about the huge number of students that failed this station, and subsequently, failed the OSPE. "There is no greater danger than underestimating your opponent" said Lao Tzu in ~540 B.C., no doubt referring to the BLS station of the OSPE.

Furthermore, ambulances within the UK respond to around 60,000 cases of suspected cardiac arrest every year, and cardiopulmonary resuscitation is only carried out in less than half of those cases.[1] The main reason for this is because the patient dies by the time the ambulance arrives.[1] There is little doubt that in many of those of cases, basic life support and CPR resuscitation performed by a bystander or household member may have saved the patient's life.

Furthermore, performing defibrillation with a semi-automated external defibrillator (AED) has been suggested to double the rate of patient survival,[2] and this something which you will be tested on in the OSPE.

This chapter will be focussed around the knowledge and skills required for BLS as outlined by the Resuscitation Council (UK), International Trauma Life Support, and the past experiences of students who succeeded in the BLS station and the OSPE as a whole.

1 The Chain of Survival for Cardiac Arrest

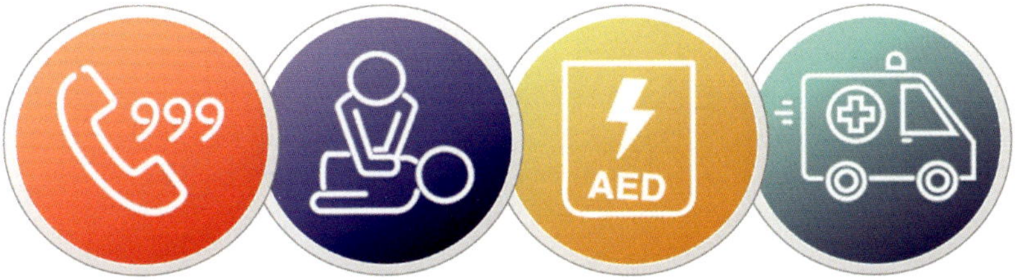

The Chain of Survival compromises of four interdependent early actions which, if considered individually and as a whole, can greatly increase the survival rate of a cardiac arrest patient outside of a clinical setting:[3,4]

1. *Early recognition and call for help*

   Recognising a cardiac arrest is crucial in enabling rapid CPR to be performed and emergency services to be alerted.[5] The common symptoms preceding cardiac arrest are tightness and an aching pain in the chest that may radiate to the arms, neck, jaw or back; nausea, heartburn, or abdominal pain; shortness of breath; cold sweat; fatigue; and light-headedness and weakness.

2. *Early bystander CPR*

   The prompt and rapid initiation of CPR by a bystander can double the chances of survival of a cardiac patient.[6]

3. *Early defibrillation*

   Semi-automated defibrillators (AED) can be widely accessed in many public areas in the UK. Most shopping malls, tube stations, schools, and public institutions will have an AED to be used in emergency situations (note that this may display as a possible question in the OSPE examination). The use of an AED within 3-5 minutes of collapsing upon the onset of cardiac arrest can improve patient survival chance by 50-70%.[7]

4. *Early advanced life support and standardised post-resuscitation care*

   Advanced life support and care by a qualified medical/paramedical team will be required in any instance of cardiac failure.

2 Performing a primary survey for life-threatening conditions

Before approaching any patient, whether that be on the ward, in a GP, or on the street before you are about to perform BLS, you must do a Primary Survey to determine if the patient has any life-threatening conditions. If you follow each step of the Primary Survey methodically, you can identify each life-threatening condition and deal with it in order of priority. A good acronym to remember for the steps of the Primary Survey is **'DRs ABC'**, which is especially useful when approaching someone collapsed on the floor:

D*anger* – is it safe to approach the patient and provide help?
R*esponse* – is the patient responding to my words/actions?
S*hout for help* – Get someone else onto the scene to help
A*irways* – is the patient's airway open and clear?
B*reathing* – is the patient breathing?
C*irculation* – is the patient severely bleeding?

1. Danger – Ensuring personal and patient safety

   Before starting any procedure, you must ensure that the safety of yourself and the patient is maintained. Injuring yourself (the first-aider) may result in you being unable to rescue the patient, and further exacerbating the problem.

   Ensure that your positioning and surroundings are not harmful, such as by being in the middle of the street; next to an ongoing fire; near exposed live electricity; or any other major threat to your health. Another key awareness is to pay attention to the number of people in need of help. In a situation where you find several people collapsed unconscious, approach with significant caution after you have called for help. Take into consideration the possibility of the existence of a mass harm causing event, such as a significant gas leak.

Good Medical Practice

Make sure to wear protective materials, such as gloves, if these are available to you, and be aware of anything sharp around you.
In fact, it is good medical practice to quickly pat the patient's pockets to make sure that nothing sharp is protruding at you. Although, take this advice with a pinch of salt, as the patient might not be unconscious and might think you're trying to steal from them.

2. Responsiveness assessment

To check the responsiveness of the patient, ask them "are you all right?", "can you hear me?", "can you open your eyes?". Make sure to project to your voice very loud.

If you receive no response here, give the patient a command: "Open your eyes!". Again, don't be afraid to project your voice.

If no response still, squeeze the patients descending trapezius muscle or ear lobule (the floppy bit at the bottom of the ear) whilst loudly asking "can you open your eyes?". This is to elicit the patient's pain response, which should wake someone up from even the deepest sleep.

An acronym to assess response is **AVPU**: **A**lert, **V**oice, **P**ain, and **U**nresponsive.

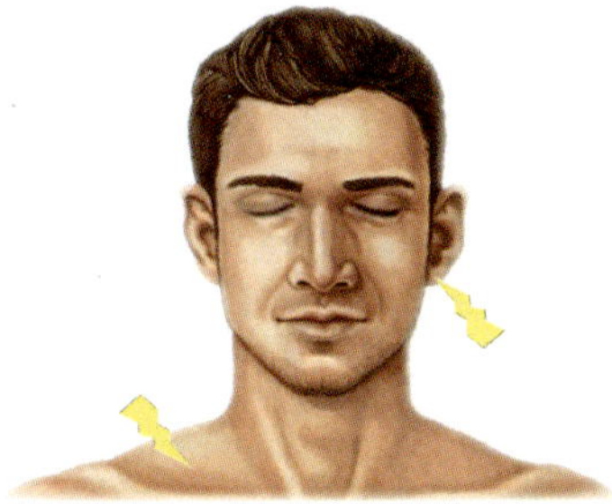

Fig 1.1 The anatomical locations to stimulate the pain response if a patient is unresponsive to a first-aiders questions and commands and seems to be unconscious.

3. Shout for help!

Should the patient not respond to the stimuli of pain, you need to shout for help in the hope of attracting a passer-by. This is essential as it will be really difficult for you to carry on by your own without any help.
Should there be a passer-by, ask them to call an ambulance.

4. Airway positioning and inspection

Use the head-tilt and chin-lift manoeuvre to open the airways in the case of tongue obstruction.[4,8] To perform this place your hand on the patient's forehead and place the tips of your fingers under the patient's chin. Then gently lift the patient's chin and open their mouth to inspect the airway for any obstructions. This could be from vomit, blood, pieces of food, their tongue, or any other object. If there is a visible obstruction which could be easily removed, try to remove it using your fingers (although this is contraindicated for the lay rescuer). While assessing and managing the patient's airway, great care should be taken to prevent excessive movement of the cervical spine.

Fig 1.2 Demonstration of the head-tilt and chin-lift manoeuvre shown on a training mannequin.

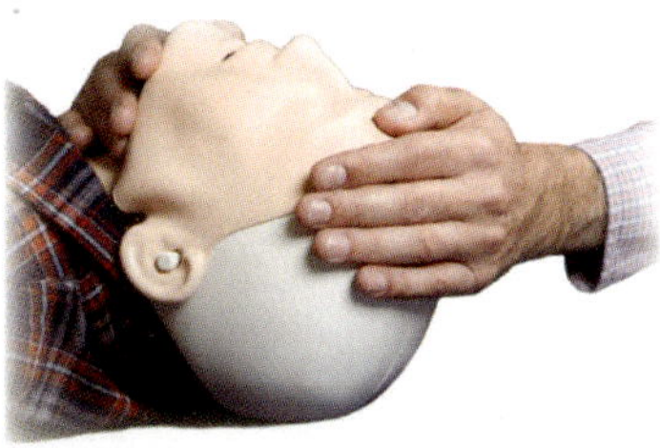

5. Breathing inspection

Keep the patient's airways open by maintaining the position of the head-tilt and chin-left manoeuvre. You must then bring your face down to the patient's face, with your cheek positioned above the patient's nose and mouth. This is to listen for any breath sounds, feel for any air expiration, and visibly observe the movements of the chest, if any.
Rising and falling of the chest is caused by the expansion and deflation of the lungs as a result of breathing. If all three signs are absent, then the patient is not breathing.
This look, listen, and feel must be done for 10 seconds.[9]

At this point, you (the first-aider) have two options on how to proceed:

1) If the patient is breathing → place them in the recovery position once you have made sure that they are not severely bleeding and continue to monitor the patient until the ambulance arrives.

   Checking for severe bleeding will be discussed in [6. Circulation] of the Primary Survey LO, and the recovery position will be discussed in LO *3 – The Recovery Position.*

2) If the patient is not breathing → initiate CPR immediately and ask a bystander to locate and bring an AED.
   CPR will be discussed in LO *4 – Cardiopulmonary Resuscitation*, and AED use will be discussed in LO *5 – Automated External Defibrillators.*

Good Medical Practice

It is important that you do not confuse agonal breaths with normal breathing. Agonal breaths are a presenting symptom within the first minutes of cardiac arrest and include slow, irregular, and deep breaths together with a wheezing sound. Indeed, agonal breaths might present in up to 40% of patients with cardiac arrest in the first minutes of the condition.[3,8]
If agonal breathing is present, you should carry on with basic life support and start CPR.

Also, the pulse can also be checked by placing two fingers over the carotid artery and feeling for its presence/absence. This is good practice once you become an experienced first-aider.

Furthermore, when asking for a bystander to call an ambulance or source an AED, it is best to be specific in your delegation of the job (i.e. by pointing and explicitly referring to a specific bystander). This is particularly important if you are surrounded by a large group of people, as we want to eliminate the bystander effect (which is an extremely interesting social psychological phenomenon that every medical student should be familiar with).

Also, when directing a bystander to get an AED, list the possible locations of where AEDs are typically found. In case you are on your own and do not have access to an AED, do not leave the patient; initiate CPR immediately.

6. Circulation

This step must only be done if the patient deemed to be breathing.
Remember, if the patient is not breathing, then immediately initiate CPR and request an AED.
If the patient is breathing, then this step is performed to assess the presence and management of severe bleeding, which is the predominant cause of post-injury deaths.

To assess for bleeding, you should gently place your hand on various locations of the patient's chest, abdomen, lower limb, upper limb, and head (particularly the hair). You must also do this on the posterior side of the patient, particularly the back, the flanks, and the back of the head. This is to feel for any blood loss and to expose it through clothing.

If the patient is bleeding, control it with your gloved hand, dressing, or clothing.
If the patient is not bleeding, then proceed with gently positioning them in the recovery position.

The pulse is also only useful for paramedical/medical staff and trained advanced first aiders.

3 The Recovery Position

The patient has to be put into recovery position if they are **1) *unconscious,* 2) *breathing,* 3) *do not have any known spinal injuries.***

Recovery position procedure:

1) Kneel by the patient's side and ensure that their legs are straight.
2) Take the patients arm closer to you and place it at a 90° angle to the patient's body, with the elbow bent and the palm of their hand facing upwards (forming a 90° angle at the elbow).
3) Take their other arm and bring it across their chest, placing the back of the hand against the cheek on the contralateral side. Maintain the patient's hand there with one arm.
4) Use your other arm to grasp the patient's leg which is farthest to you, and pull it up until it is bent at the knee while their foot is still on the floor*.
5) At this point, you are using one hand to hold the patient's hand against their cheek, and your other hand is holding the knee of the leg which you have pulled up. Now gently pull their knee until they have rolled over towards you.
6) Bring this leg in front of the body so that it is resting on the floor and helping the patient maintain balance.
7) In order to maintain the airways of the patient, gently raise the patient's chin and tilt their head back. Furthermore, to avoid choking from liquid material, make sure the face of the patient is slightly facing downwards so that the liquid can drain out from their mouth. Make sure you check that he is breathing normally, and should this stop, then immediately initiate CPR.

Note: Although these are the defined guidelines by almost every professional body within the field of resuscitation and first-aid, I find it much easier to do *Step 4* before *Step 3*.
By doing this, I am free to use both hands when lifting up the patient's leg (in case it's a rather heavy leg), and I have the flexibility to reach over to grab the patient's knee (in case they are rather tall). In fact, if I really don't have the ability to reach over and grab the patient's knee, I have the ability to move closer to it without having to commit my entire body to hold the patient's hand on their cheek.
Once I have bent the patient's knee (*Step 4*), I then go back to *Step 3* and bring the patients hand to their contralateral cheek.

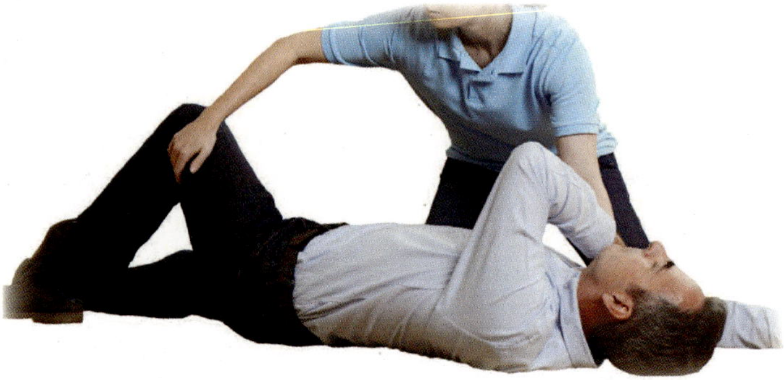

Fig 1.3 A a first-aider placing an unconscious patient in the recovery position.

4 Cardiopulmonary resuscitation

Cardiopulmonary resuscitation (CPR) is an emergency procedure that is done when a patient is unconscious and not breathing. As mentioned, when no breathing is detected in the primary survey of an unconscious patient, CPR should be started immediately.
CPR is done in an effort to manually preserve brain function until further measures are taken to restore spontaneous blood circulation and breathing in a person who is in cardiac arrest.

CPR Initiation

CPR combines chest compressions with artificial ventilation in a methodical manner.
In an adult, you begin by providing 30 chest compressions, followed by 2 rescue breaths.
This must be constantly repeated until the end of CPR.

In a child, you begin with 5 rescue breaths, followed by 30 chest compressions and 2 rescue breaths in a repeating manner. This must be constantly repeated until the end of CPR.

Chest Compressions

1) Ensure that the patient is lying on their back on a flat and hard surface.
2) Kneel by the side of the patient and place the heel of your dominant hand in the centre of the patient's chest, (in the lower half of the sternum, which in a male would roughly be between the nipples).
3) Place the heel of your less dominant hand on the hand already on the patient's sternum and interlock the fingers of your two hands.
4) Maintain straight arms and begin to compress the patient's chest to a depth of 5-6cm, which is 1/3 the chest wall depth.[10,11] Ensure that you are using your body weight to compress the chest, and you are not bending your elbows. This is done by placing your shoulders directly above your arms and the sternum.
5) Do not detach your hands from the chest of the patient after each compression, but make sure you fully decompress before beginning a new compression cycle.[12]
6) Maintain a rate of 100-120 compressions per minute to allow sufficient circulation.
7) Perform a cycle of 30 chest compressions and 2 rescue breaths, while you await an AED.

Note: Chest compressions are the most important part of CPR, and although rescue breaths are extremely effective, they are not a necessity. Also, the effectiveness of chest compressions is from the technique more so than the quantity. Make sure you have a good technique and are compressing & decompressing effectively.

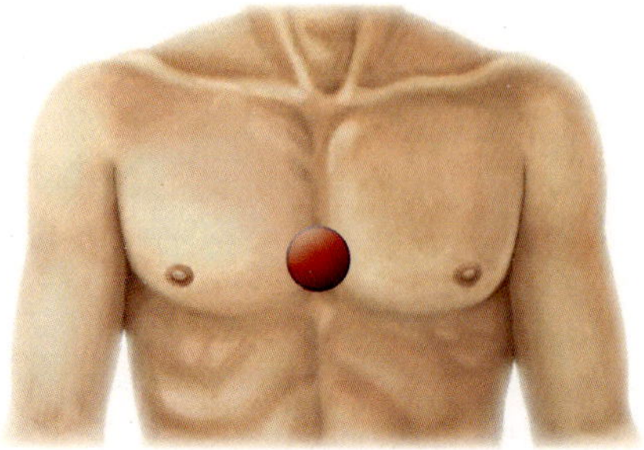

Fig 1.4 The location on the chest where the chest compressions should take place for CPR.

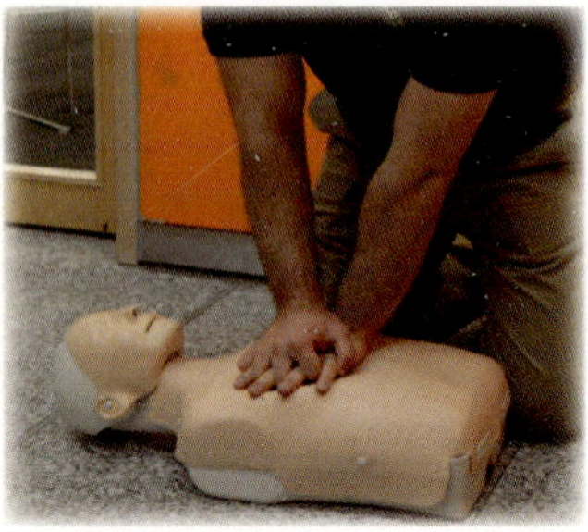

Fig 1.5 The correct technique for doing chest compressions, as demonstrated on a training mannequin.

Artificial Ventilation

1) After 30 chest compressions are performed, initiate 2 rescue breaths.
2) Use the head-tilt and chin-lift manoeuvre to open the patient's mouth and airways.
3) Pinch the patient's nostrils, and position your mouth on top of, and around the patient's mouth. Ensure that you have created a tight seal between your mouth and the patients.
4) Blow with slowly but with relative force into the patient's mouth. The duration of each rescue breath should be ~1 second.
5) After each breath, immediately observe for the patient's chest to rise and fall. Make sure to stop pinching the patient's nose and maintain the head-tilt and chin-lift positioning.
6) Take a deep breath and perform another rescue breath before proceeding onto the chest compressions.

Note: Do not interrupt chest compressions for more than 10 seconds. As mentioned, chest compressions are the most important part of CPR. Also, the use of mouth-to-mouth ventilation is limited in a clinical setting due to the risk of infection transmission. If the patient has a known potentially transmittable infection, then it is better to only perform repeated chest compressions.

Halting CPR

CPR should be maintained until:

1) A senior health professional instructs you to halt.
2) You become exhausted, in which case CPR should be resumed by a bystander.
3) The patient has been resuscitated, in which case consider the recovery position if they are still unresponsive.
4) Upon the verbal instructions of an AED.

5 Automated External Defibrillators (AED)

Once an AED arrives, immediately attach the two electrode pads to the patient, one on the right of the sternum below the clavicle and the on the left mid-axillary line below the breast level on the chest wall, as shown in ***Fig 1.6***. In the case that more than one rescuer is present, CPR should be continued whilst the electrodes are being placed on the patient.

The electrodes must be placed firmly on a patient's skin, so all obstructive clothing must be removed, and excessive hair shaved off. Scissors and a razor blade are provided in the AED pack for this purpose. Chest piercings must also be removed to avoid burns with the defibrillator. Furthermore, instructive diagrams on where to place the electrodes are given on the electrode pads.

Once you have attached the electrodes and pressed the clearly defined on-button to initiate the AED, follow the audio-visual instructions given and only interrupt chest compressions when asked to do so by the AED. Usually, the AED will notify you that it is analysing the rhythm of the patient, at which point chest compressions must be STOPPED, all touching of the patient must cease immediately.

The two outcomes that follow are:

1) Shock is indicated by the AED. Make sure that no one is touching the patient during this time by shouting: "Everyone stand clear of the patient!" and physically clearing the area above the patient with your arms.

2) Kneel by the side of the patient and place the heel of your less dominant hand in the centre of the patient's chest, (in the lower half of the sternum, which in a male would roughly be between the nipples).

Medical Fact

Paediatric patients have one electrode pad placed on the anterior part of the chest, left of the sternum, and the other is placed on their back.

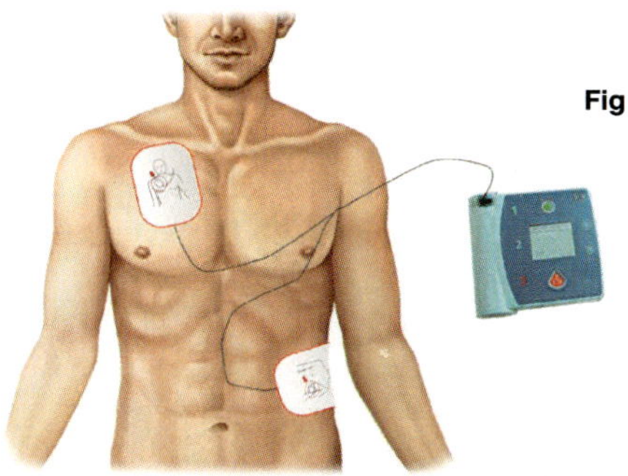

Fig 1.6 The active locations of the electrode pads as described by the depicted AED.

6 First-aid in a choking emergency

Chocking is a very common life-threatening situation, and early intervention has the potential to save the life of the patient. Therefore, it is crucial to know first aid surrounding choking.

Before first aid intervention, it is essential to assess the severity of chocking:

Mild airway obstruction

In a mild chocking situation caused by a partial airway obstruction, one must simply encourage coughing. Indeed, any other intervention other than the encouragement of coughing in a patient with a partial airway obstruction might worsen their situation and lead to a complete airway obstruction. Keep the patient under continuous observation to see if the situation deteriorates into complete airway obstruction or whether the situation is relieved.

Severe airway obstruction

In the situation in which there is a severe/complete airway obstruction, and coughing is ineffective, the first aider must start physical intervention. It begins with 5 back blows.

Back blow procedure: You have to stand behind the patient, using one hand to support the chest whilst they lean forward. Using the heel of your other hand, give five firm blows in a slightly upward direction on the back of the patient between the scapulae.
Should the back blows be ineffective, give the patient 5 abdominal thrusts.

Abdominal thrust procedure: Stand directly behind the patient whilst they lean slightly forward and wrap your arms around the upper abdomen, slightly below the transpyloric plane. Clench a fist with your predominant hand and grab this with your other hand. Position your clenched hands between the umbilicus and the xiphoid process and firmly pull inwards and upwards.
Repeat this procedure 5 times. If there is no relief, then repeat with the five back blows.[13,14]

If the choking escalates into to the patient becoming unresponsive, immediately begin the Primary Survey and appropriate CPR/recovery position after alerting the emergency services.

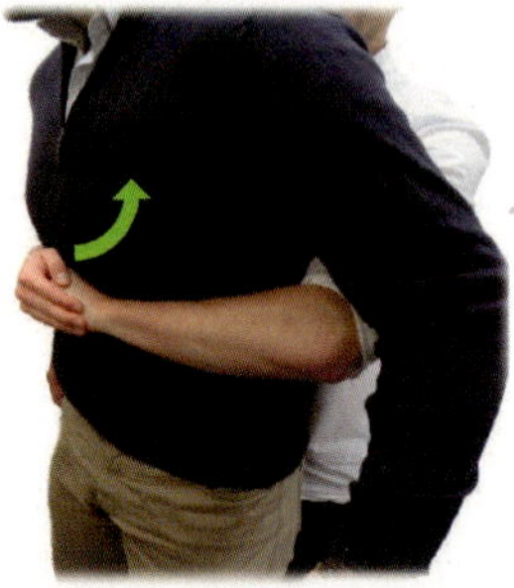

Fig 1.7 The abdominal thrusts procedure.

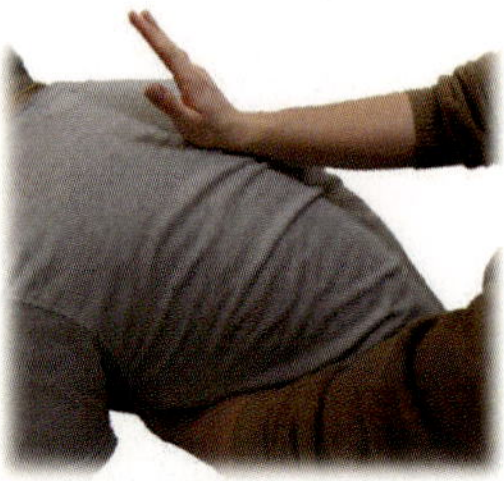

Fig 1.8 The back blow procedure.

Clinical Communication

By Junzheng Wang

Introduction to the chapter

Since the age of paternalistic medicine, clinical communications have come a long way towards being patient-centred, and a two-way exchange of information between the clinician and the patient. No longer are patients viewed simply as problems to be fixed with scalpels or pills, with their opinions, beliefs, and views largely irrelevant. We have come to the realisation that co-production and partnership working leads to better outcomes if we fully involve patients in the decision-making process and engage them in their own care.

Good communication with patients helps to reduce anxiety, and through encouraging patients to take an active part in the conversation, build confidence to feel valued, respected and cared for as a stakeholder in control of their own healthcare. This is so important as patients must not feel institutionalised by "the system", losing any say they had over their own lives to a depersonalised entity once they fall ill, eventually leading to poorer outcomes.

This chapter will seek to capture the key points, skills and techniques to help you secure the clinical communication marks through ensuring your physical examinations and history taking in the OSPE is more than simply fulfilling a textbook checklist, but truly patient-centred, orientated towards the needs, experiences and feelings of the individual in front of you.

Clinical communications will be assessed within the summative OSPE in two ways:

1. A dedicated station within the 7-station circuit to take a focussed history with a simulated patient. The format will be identical to your previous in-course formative simulated patient sessions and will be based entirely on what has been covered in the course.

2. Clinical Communications will also be examined within all other stations; including your introductions upon entering the station, respect and empathy towards the patient throughout, and your conclusion at the end.

For all stations

These general points apply to all OSPE stations and will help you make a good impression on both the patient and the examiner. These skills are also assessed, and should be relatively easy marks to gain!

1.1 Dress code

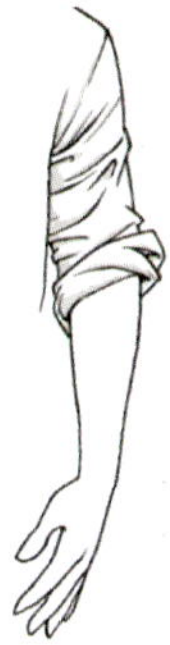

Impressions matter, so it is important that you appear professional at all times during the exam. Smart dress with rolled up sleeves and bare below the elbow; wristwatch should be removed but can be secured around your belt/belt loop. Alternatively, it is a good idea to invest in a fob watch.

Please do not wear any shoes which leave the toes exposed.
This is not allowed in a clinical setting and will not be allowed in the OSPE.

1.2 Entering the station

Outside each station, you will have 1 minute to read an introductory brief before entering, which will include the patient's name, their date of birth, and what you need to do inside.

1. **Greet both the patient and examiner, and state your name and candidate number:**
   A simple "hello", or "good morning/afternoon" will suffice, before proceeding to give your name and candidate number to the examiner.
   "My name is Jane Smith and my candidate number is 8919."

   A smile goes a long way! Be positive and leave a great first impression.

2. **Introduce yourself to the patient, and check their name and DoB:**
   Don't be afraid to repeat some things you have just said to the examiner, as it is vital that you introduce yourself properly to the patient to build that initial rapport and understanding, as well as checking that you are with the correct patient.
   "Hi there. My name Jane Smith, and I am a second-year medical student at Imperial College London. Can I please confirm your name and date of birth?"

3. **Explain your task:**
   Explain to the patient clearly, using everyday language without medical jargon, what you will be doing, whether it is to take a history, or performing an examination.
   Avoid technical terminology such as thorax, auscultate, and palpate; use 'chest'; listen to'; and 'feel for' instead.

You should also warn the patient if you require them to be undressed in some way in order to perform the physical examination - be very clear in what you are going to do and what you require from the patient before you ask for their consent.

"I have been asked by the doctor to examine your chest, which will involve having a general look, before tapping on your chest and having a listen to your breathing. To do this I would need you to take your top off and expose your chest area if that's okay with you?"

4. **Obtain consent:**
   You must explicitly gain consent from the patient before you perform any examination/start taking the history.
   Normally you would ask the patient if they would like a chaperone to be present, in the case of the OSPE exam, you would simply state that the examiner would act as the chaperone.

   "... I have been asked to examine your abdomen, which will involve... is this okay? The examiner will act as the chaperone for this examination."

5. **Pain or discomfort?**
   Always ask the patient if they are in any pain or discomfort before going ahead with any examination.
   You should tell the patient that they should let you know if they feel any pain during the examination.

   "Do you have any pain or discomfort anywhere?" ... "Please let me know if you start feeling any pain during the examination."

6. **Position the bed angle:**
   The patient should be positioned at a 45° angle for cardiology and respiratory examinations.
   An abdominal exam should be conducted with the patient lying flat.
   Usually, the bed is already adjusted in the OSPE, but don't just blindly count on this.

7. **Hand hygeine:**
   Very important for infection control, and a very easy mark in the exam. You should gel your hands before and after touching the patient to avoid cross-contamination.

   Look for the hand sanitiser as you enter the station. If you can't find it, ask the examiner where it is. Also, don't forget to sanitise your hands again before you examine the patient if you had to adjust the bed.

Example scenario:

1. Enter the HNS station.
   > To the examiner: *"Good morning, my name is Jane Smith, candidate number is 8919".*
2. Examiner greets you, may tell you what is required of you, and says: *"you may proceed."*
3. > To the patient - *"Hi, my name is Jane, a second-year medical student at Imperial College London. Can I confirm your name and your date of birth please?"*
4. Patient gives name and DoB.
   "Thank you. I've been asked today to examine your head, neck, and spine, which will involve me asking you to do a range of movements and having a feel of your neck.
   Would that be ok?"
5. Patient consents.
   "Thank you, are you in any pain or discomfort at all?"
   "Would you be able to sit up on the side of the bed for me?"
6. Sanitise your hands

1.3 During the station

Polite, respectful, and maintain transparency of conduct.

Think "**PAT**"

Permission: "Can you lie down for me please?" "Would you mind...."
Assessment procedure
Thanks: Always thank the patient after each action. "Okay, thank you".

Demonstration
Demonstrate the action or movement you want the patient to perform if required to ensure the patient is clear on what you are asking them to do. For example, *"could you raise your arm for me".*

Exposure
If you need to request the patient to remove clothing for an examination, always be clear in your request and explain why this is necessary.

"Can you remove your top for me please so that I can look at.... I am going to have a feel of..." etc.

Once the patient's examination is over, tell the patient they can put their item of clothing back on. Do not leave the patient without clothing whilst you continue with the examiner's questions, and offer to help the patient re-dress if appropriate.

Be conscious of the distance between you and the patient - this should be always appropriate according to what you are doing. You should maintain appropriate eye contact/body positioning, particularly when conducting an examination.

Empathetic
Use appropriate verbal and non-verbal behaviours to build rapport with the patient, for example:

- Avoiding excessive 'ums' and 'errs' when speaking to the patient.
- Show sensitivity toward the patient, especially when touching them.
- Pick up verbal and non-verbal cues - use appropriate tone, speed and volume of voice in response to patient cues, for example, if someone seems distracted by other concerns.
- Notice and acknowledge a patient who suddenly winces in pain or shows other expressions or signs of discomfort during physical examinations.

1.4 Concluding the station

When you have finished examining the patient, don't forget to thank them and ask them if they require assistance getting dressed. Also, don't forget to sanitise your hands after dealing with a patient.

Described here are the general LO's for every single station and you should absolutely master these skills. Not only are they easy marks but they are crucial throughout your medical career. Remember, the mark of a good doctor is one who patients know by name.

The Clinical Communication station

The aim of this station is to take a focussed history with the simulated patient, which examines your knowledge of what to cover during a patient interview (the content elements) and your skills in obtaining the necessary information sensitively and professionally through using appropriate questions, a logical structure, and paying attention to verbal and non-verbal cues (the process elements). The exam is designed to test how effective you are able to integrate content with process.

There are no specific, set orders to how the interview should be structured - treat it as a natural conversation, but make sure the conversation is ordered logically.

2.1 Outside the station

You will have 1 minute to read the background information outside the station before the 10 minutes you will have inside to conduct the interview.

The background information tends to read along the lines of: "You have been asked by the GP to take a history from patient *X*, DOB *dd/mm/yyyy* before their consultation. You have 10 minutes."

2.2 Introducing yourself

As for any OSPE station, you should greet patient and examiner; introduce yourself, your role, and why you are there; and gain their consent for proceeding with the interview.

Explain clearly the purpose of the interview and obtain consent: "The GP has asked me to speak with you for 10 minutes to take your history before your consultation, which I will then feedback to the doctor. Is this okay with you?"

To reassure the patient, you can mention that anything they mention will remain confidential and that you will relay everything you have discussed back to the doctor at the end of the interview.

(Yes) → "Is it okay if I take a seat" *(Yes)*

Check the name and DOB:
"Before we continue, can I just confirm your name and date of birth."

2.3 Opening the conversation

Take your time and don't rush the conversion. You will have 10 minutes, which should be ample time to explore each content element (see below).

Begin with some generic open questions, and then let the patient speak:

- *"How are you feeling this morning?"*
- *"So what brought you into the clinic today?"*

You will find that often simple open questions like this will prompt the patient to tell you their ***Presenting Complaint*** **(PC)**:

For example *"Oh I'm been feeling awful since I woke up this morning, I just can't stop coughing really badly"* - which you can then explore further:

- *"Can you tell me more about it?"*
- Clarify anything which you might not be sure about - *"dizzy - do you mean feeling lightheaded or is the room spinning around you?"*

Beware that there could be more than one presenting complaint.

- Give the patient an opportunity to add anything else at the end: "Okay, so you have told me about the cough, fever, and migraines. Are there any other symptoms you would like to tell me before we continue?"

However, It is important to note that everyone will respond slightly differently to questions, for example not everyone will open up immediately following your initial open question and tell you everything.

Some patients might only give a short one-line answer for 10 seconds after the first question and another might talk for a whole minute. This is especially the case with simulated patient actors who have been given specific instructions on how easily they should reveal information.

If your initial open question does not elicit as much information as you would have liked, do not panic, and jump to a closed question straight away. Continue asking some more open questions, perhaps more focussed on what the patient has just told you.

Remember, a degree of mental flexibility is always required! Remember there is no fixed "recipe" as to how you go about taking the history, as long as you gather all the information required by the end.

Summarising and signposting
Signal clearly to the patient that you are moving onto the next section, and signpost so that the patient understands what is going on and why it is relevant:

"So, to help me get a better understanding of what's going on, I am now going to ask you some more questions about each of the symptoms which you've just told me about, if that's okay?"

Don't interrupt the patient
Otherwise, you may cut them off before they explain fully and miss a vital piece of information.

Build rapport with patient by being empathetic and observant of verbal and non-verbal cues
For example, if you can see the patient is in physical discomfort, show empathy and concern by asking something along the lines of *"How are you feeling this morning? Are you alright, because I can see that you are..."*

Be aware of your body language, for example maintaining eye contact. Ensure you have an open posture, but make sure you don't cross your arms as it indicates a closure from your side.
Don't fiddle or fidget with anything.

Also, use verbal cues to show empathy, understanding, and encouragement for the patient to continue, for example, *"I understand that this must be really stressful for you, but we will do our best to take care of you..."*

The beginning of the station could be considered the most important bit. However, if you do not manage to start in the best way, do not stress out too much, carry on the consultation and if there is anything you missed to ask or do, politely ask later on.

2.4 Exploring further

In this section, we will be addressing the ***History of Presenting Complaint*** **(HPC)** and other elements about the patient's medical background.

Use the "question cone" technique
Start with more open questions such as *"what brought you into the clinic today?"* then gradually shift to more closed questions as you focus in on specific aspects.

- *"So, can you tell me a bit more about it?"*
- *"Can you describe it for me?"*
- *"When did the symptom start?"*
- *"Have you had it before?", "Are there any difference?" "Any previous investigations or treatments?"*

Note that to effectively integrate content and process, often you will need to move between open and closed questions rather than simply moving from a more open to a closed direction.

For pain, think about SOCRATES

- **Site** - *"where exactly is the pain?"*
  Ask them to point to it to make it clearer for you.
- **Onset** - *"when did the pain start?", "Did it come about suddenly or gradually?"*
- **Character** - *"can you describe the pain for me?", "Is it sharp? Dull? Stabbing? Aching? etc..."*
- **Radiation** - "does the pain spread to anywhere else on the body or is it in a specific location?"
- **Associated** - "Any other symptoms which you may have noticed?"
- **Time** - "does the pain develop during particular times of the day?"
- **Exacerbating or relieving factors** - "does anything make the pain better or worse?"
- **Scale** - "on a scale of 1 - 10, with 10 being the worst pain you can possibly imagine, how would you score the pain you've experienced/or are experiencing?"

Although this framework is tailored to the description of pain, many aspects (e.g. site, onset, time, exacerbating factors) could be adapted for other symptoms too, for example, a cough.

- *When did the cough start?*
- *How would you describe it? Dry? Chesty?*
- *Any other symptoms? Sputum? Wheeze? SOB?*
- *Does anything make the cough better/worse?*

Note: the patient might even tell you some of these pieces of information at the start of the conversation when talking about the presenting complaints, in which case you can simply ask if the information you have already gained regarding the pain is correct and then move on to ask any missing parts.

Integrate ICE within your interview

- **Ideas:** *"Do you have any ideas as to what might be causing your cough?" "What do you think might be causing these symptoms?" "How do you think this may have started?"*
- **Concerns**: *"Is there anything in particular that you're worried about?"*
- ***Expectations:*** "What are you hoping the doctor will do for you today?" "What would be the best outcome for you from your perspective?"

Of course, you do not have to ask about all three elements together. Try to integrate them with your other questions and keep to the natural flow of the conversation, but do make sure you address ICE within your interview. For example, the patient's concerns could link to previous medical conditions or their family history.

Remember to respond appropriately and supportively, especially when the patient tells you about their concerns which they may feel self-conscious about, so it is important that you show empathy and encourage them to continue.

You may also want to follow up on symptoms with a relevant system review here rather than towards the end. For example, if the patient presents with chest pain, you can ask the patient if they have any other cardiac or respiratory symptom, see **2.8** - *System review.*

2.5 Past Medical History (PMH) and Drug History (DHx)

You should find out if the patient has any other medical conditions, either present or in the past, along with any medications they currently take and any allergies.

Past Medical History (PMH)

- *"Can I ask if you have any other medical conditions?"*
- *"Have you had any medical problems in the past?"*

Note that often patients may not tell you straight away about something which they may have had 10 years ago or in childhood, which they may consider to be not relevant to the present situation but could actually be important. To elicit this information, emphasise with *"Have you ever..."*.

- *"Have you ever been admitted to hospital?"*
- *"Have you ever had any surgeries?"*

Keep the questions open as the patient will often tell you information about their past medical history which you will want to know without any further prompts, for example with our cough patient:

- *"Can I ask if you have any other medical conditions?"*
- *"Yes, I was diagnosed with diabetes a few years ago but I'm on top of it with my daily metformin tablets, insulin injections and diet planning."*

If they are not more forthcoming, for example, by simply stating *"Yes, I also have diabetes"*, you can ask some follow up questions such as:

- *"And how are you managing your diabetes?"*
- *"How long ago were you diagnosed?"*
- *"Do you have any other medical issues other than your diabetes?"*

Again, apply the question cone technique as appropriate. Note that you are not expected to ask closed questions - however, if there are any past medical history which is particularly relevant to the patient's presenting complaint, it may be worth following up with some further questions to identify information which would only be given when prompted.

Drug History (DHx)

It's very important to find out if they are taking any medications, especially if they have previously mentioned that they have an existing medical condition. Also, patients often neglect to mention any over the counter (OTC) drugs such as paracetamol, ibuprofen, or antacids, unless you explicitly ask.

- *"Are you currently taking any medications?"*
- *"Are you currently taking any medications bought over the counter?"*
    - > If yes, what for? Dose and frequency?
    - > When started?
    - > Any side effects?
    - > Any compliance issues?
        - > If yes, *"Do you have any problems with taking your medication?" "Do you ever miss a dose?"*

Allergies

- *"Do you suffer from any allergies?"*
- *"Are you aware if you are allergic to any medications?"*

2.6 Family History (FHx)

Often family history can be a sensitive topic, so again it is vital that you approach this with empathy in mind and keep questions relevant.

- *"Would you mind if I ask about any medical conditions which run in the family?"*
- If the patient has a respiratory condition for example - *"Can I ask if there is a family history of respiratory problems?"*

Of course, this could come up in the middle of the PMH section, or when you ask the patient about their concerns. For example, the patient may divulge that they are concerned that their chest pain could indicate heart problems because several close relatives all passed away due to heart attacks. *"I'm sorry to hear that..."*

You could also ask whether they think their condition might be family related, linking to the ideas component of ICE.

- *"Do you think this might be family related, or have anything to do with the family history?"*

2.7 Social History (SHx)

Lifestyle factors - smoking, alcohol, substance misuse, occupation, travel

Smoking and alcohol are major lifestyle risk factors which we want to ask every patient.

- *"Can I ask if you smoke?*
- *"Can I ask if you drink at all?"*

If the answer is yes, then we want to know on average, how many cigarettes the patient smokes, or how many units does the patient drink per week.

- If the patient does not know how many units of alcohol they consume on an average week, you can ask for the actual alcohol they drink and how often, for example, *"a glass of wine everyday day at dinner".*

With smoking, ask:

- *"How long have you been smoking for?"*
- *"Have you ever smoked? If so when did you stop? How much did you used to smoke?"* This question is important as an ex-smoker can answer "no" to *"do you smoke?".*

Be sensitive around asking the patient if they have used recreational drugs. Normalise the question by stating "this is a standard question we have to ask all patients" before asking:

- *Would you mind telling me if you use, or have ever used recreational drugs?"*
  > If yes, *"Would you mind me asking what drugs? How often/long/much?"*

Occupation could also be important to a patient's history, whether it may be a source of stress, for example high workload, or the patient may be concerned about missing work, or a risk factor for their medical condition.

- *"What do you do for a living?"*

Our cough patient may tell you that he is a builder working for a demolition company specialising in asbestos removal – in which case this is a highly relevant risk factor.
Or, he might disclose to you that he has a large family to support on his own and is really worried the impact of missing work for an extended period of time.

- Also think about previous jobs.
- Again, be sympathetic and supportive as appropriate.

Travel history may also be relevant to some patients:

- *"Have you been abroad anywhere recently?"*
- *"Did you fall ill at all during the trip?"*
- *"Did you take any vaccines?" etc.*

Homelife/family situation might be a source of worry for some patients, for example, if they have children at home, but no one else to look after them if the patient is ill. The impacts on the person's daily life could also be covered before this section.

- *"Is there anyone else at home?"*
- *"Do you live with anyone at home?"*
- *"Do you have any dependents at home?"*
- *"Do you have any pets?"*
- How is the PC impacting their life? How has it affected their daily living?

Mobility and functional ability – this is especially for elderly patients, and links into the last point above about how does the PC impact on their everyday life.

Think about if they need, and have support at home e.g. carers, family support?

- Where do they live and are they mobile, for example, if they have difficulty walking but live on the second floor, climbing stairs will be an issue.
- Can they exercise – if difficult, what is their exercise tolerance?
- Do they drive? Can they leave home easily and regularly?

Sexual history - again be sensitive and ask only if relevant

Diet – if relevant to PC/PMH

- *"Would you say you have a healthy diet?"*
- *"Can you take me through a typical day's food and drink?"*
- *"Can I ask you about your weight?" "Do you have any concerns over your weight?"* •
- *"Do you eat a special diet?"* If yes, what and why?

2.8 Systems review

Often you will have covered a lot of the relevant symptoms in sections before this and will have integrated it within your conversation - for example, the patient might tell you that when he coughed there was sputum. At that point, you might naturally decide to explore the systems review by asking if it was related to anything else, if there was blood in the sputum etc. before continuing.

Remember you are not expected to cover all of this fully, so there is no need to spend a lot of time on this section. In fact, the systems review is mostly relevant to your clinical years, but we've decided to include it as a reference for the future. Also, remember this is not a comprehensive list!

Remember to keep any questions focussed and relevant to the PC.

- *"Do you have any problems with..."*
- *"Have you experienced any..."*

General questions (particularly relevant for cancer or TB):
1. weight loss
2. night sweats
3. any lumps
4. fatigue
5. appetite
6. fevers
7. itch
8. recent trauma

CVS and respiratory systems:
1. chest pain (think SOCRATES), palpitations
2. exertional dyspnoea (quantify exercise tolerance: how many stairs)
3. paroxysmal nocturnal dyspnoea
4. breathless on lying flat (orthopnoea, a symptom of left ventricular failure)
5. oedema
6. cough or wheeze
7. sputum
8. haemoptysis (coughing up blood)

Gastrointestinal
1. abdominal pain (think SOCRATES)
2. nausea/vomiting
3. vomiting blood (haematemesis)
4. indigestion;
5. stool – colour, consistency, blood
6. melaena - passing altered (black) blood
7. tenesmus (feeling that there is something in the rectum that cannot be passed e.g. due to a tumour)

Neurology

1. sensory changes in sight/hearing/smell/taste
2. dizziness, fainting, seizures
3. poor balance
4. headache
5. speech disturbances
6. pins and needles (paraesthesia), numbness
7. muscle weakness "Do your arms and legs work?"
8. sphincter disturbance
9. higher mental function and psychiatric symptoms

Genitourinary/renal

1. incontinence
2. painful urination (dysuria), blood in urine (haematuria), need to pass urine at night (nocturia), frequent need to pass urine (polyuria), any offensive odour?
3. hesitancy, terminal dribbling
4. menstruation - frequency, regularity, heavy or light, duration, painful, first day of last menstrual period.
5. number of pregnancies
6. possibility of current pregnancy?
7. menarche, menopause

Musculoskeletal

1. joint pain
2. stiffness
3. swelling

2.9 Summary and conclusion

Signal that the interview is drawing to a close by giving a concise summary of the interview:

- *"Thank you very much for speaking to me today, so before we finish I would just like to quickly summarise what you have just told me..."*
- Keep your summary concise, making sure to note the key points from the interview.

Invite the patient to contribute any additional information which they may have not yet told you or that you have missed.

- *"Would you agree that is an accurate summary of what you have been telling me? Is there anything else which I may have missed, or you would like to add for me to mention back to the GP?"*
- *"Before I leave, is there anything else you would like me to pass on to the GP?"*
- *"Do you have any questions for me to take back to your GP for you?*

If you realise at this point that you have missed something:

- *Clarify that you have forgotten and then ask the question.*
- *Always better to ask and get the necessary information than to not find out.*

Thank the patient at the end.

Final remarks

Use signposting to clearly signal to the patient that you are moving on to another section of the history. Quickly summarise what the patient has just told you, and link into what you want to talk about next. "Okay, so you have just told me... and now I would just like to move on to..."

These mini summaries can also help you gain a brief moment of time to pull your thoughts together if you suddenly forget what next to say or talk about.

Build rapport with the patient, if they mention for example that they are concerned about falling ill because they have two young children at home, a simple question like *"how old are they?"* or *"what are their names?"* helps to build that personal connection with the patient, and shows that you are taking a genuine interest in their narrative.

Respond to non-verbal cues as well as verbal cues. If the patient looks worried, comment on it empathetically - *"you look concerned - is there anything which worries you?"*

There are no specific, set orders to how the interview should be structured - treat it as a natural conversation, but make sure the conversation is ordered logically.

Best of luck in your exams.

The Respiratory System

By Seungmin Han

Introduction to the chapter

The respiratory station can be one of the less challenging stations if you have sound knowledge of the surface anatomy around the chest. Having said that, it is not to be neglected as it is a key station in the OSPEs and introduces techniques that are clinically very relevant. The idea of auscultation through an instrument was established by René Laennec in the 19th century; he found that compared to the traditional auscultation, where a physician's ear would be placed directly on to the patient's chest, indirect auscultation improved clarity of the chest sounds – the stethoscope at the time was a rolled-up paper cone.

The development of percussion as a part of the physical examination dates to 18th century, but it is said that the principles of both auscultation and percussion had been practised since the Egyptian times. Such techniques have developed significantly since its first use and are still used frequently in clinical settings. This station will equip you with a solid foundation of knowledge to perform these techniques and prepare you for application to clinical cases.

This chapter is structured so that it takes you through the anatomy-related then the practical learning objectives, where you can apply the technique and knowledge together. There are some suggested phrases you could use in the exam, which is indicated in italic writing. Remember, these are only suggestions and as you practice, try and develop your own way of communication that suit you best – this will be easier for you than learning phrases off by heart.

Clinical Communication

"I have been asked to perform a chest examination on you, and this involves me tapping on different parts of your chest and listening to your breathing using my stethoscope. I would need you to have your chest exposed for that and the examiner will act as your chaperone. Is that okay with you?"

Abbreviations

- AML: anterior midline
- MCL: midclavicular line
- MAL: mid-axillary line
- PML: posterior median line
- CC: costal cartilage
- ICS: intercostal space

Fig 3.1 The lungs in situ.

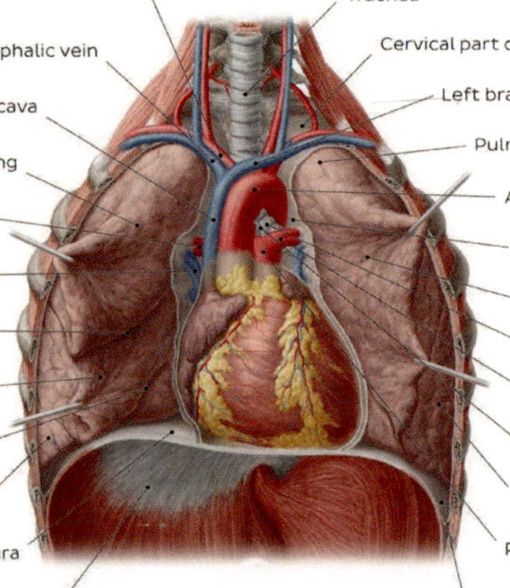

1 Identify the bones and landmarks of the chest wall

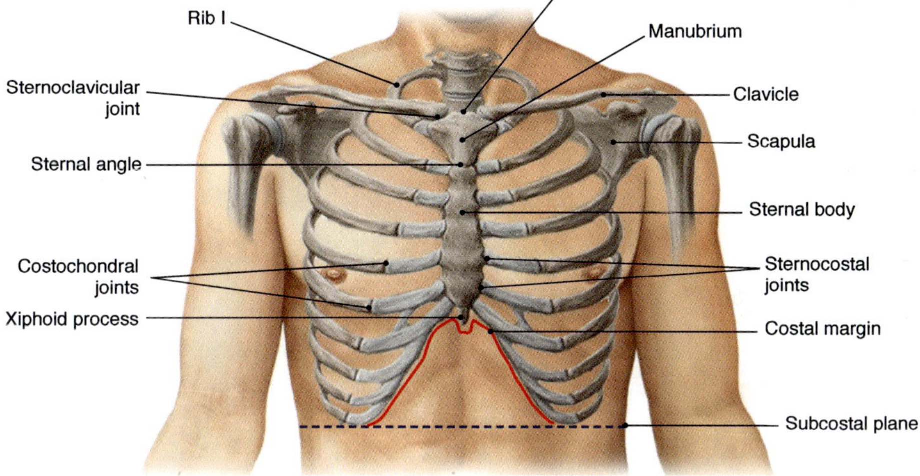

Fig 3.2 The bones, landmarks and margins of the ventral chest wall.

The sternum is a superficial flat bone consisting of the manubrium, the sternal body, and the xiphisternum (xiphoid process) and it forms the midline of the ventral skeletal trunk. It's functions are to protect vital thoracic organs and vessels from trauma, to act as the bony attachment for various muscles of the body, and to form the ribcage through it's seven sternocostal joints with the costal cartilages of ribs I - VII (known as the true ribs). All the sternocostal joints are synovial joints, apart from the first, which is a synarthrosis.

Ribs VIII - X are known as false ribs, as they attach indirectly to the sternum through the costal cartilage of rib VII, and ribs XI and XII are floating ribs, as they do not attach to the sternum.

The subcostal plane is at the level of L3 vertebra, and it is a plane passing through the lowest margin of the ribs. This plane is of particular significance when dividing the abdomen into regions for examination.

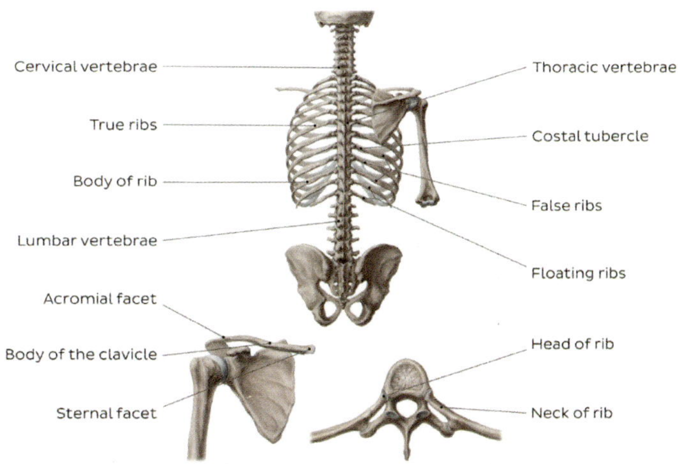

Fig 3.3 The bones of the dorsal chest wall.

2 The surface markings of the lobes of the right and left lungs

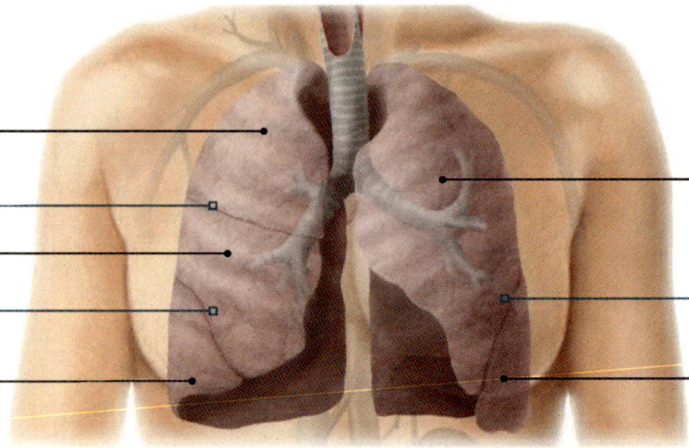

Fig 3.4 The lungs in situ, with the lobes and fissures labelled. The left lung only has one fissure separating its two lobes, and a significant cardiac depression. The right lung has two fissures separating its three lobes.

Right lung

Upper lobe

Apex is 2-3cm above medial third of right clavicle → sternoclavicular joint → right 2nd CC which is lateral to sternal angle → 4th right CC → T3 just lateral to PML → T1 just lateral to PML

Middle lobe

4th right CC → 6th right CC just lateral to AML → 6th rib at MCL → 4th rib at MAL

Lower lobe

6th right CC just lateral to AML → 6th rib at MCL → 8th rib at MAL → 10th rib at scapular line → 10th rib at just lateral to PML

Left lung

Upper lobe

Apex is 2-3cm above medial third of left clavicle → sternoclavicular joint → left 2nd CC, which is lateral to sternal angle → 4th CC → 6th CC lateral to AML → T3 just lateral to PML → T1 just lateral to PML

Lower lobe

6th left rib at MCL → 8th rib at MAL → 10th rib at scapular line → 10th rib at just lateral to PML

At roughly 4th to 6th rib level anteriorly, the left lung deviates from the midline, compared to the right lung, due to the heart's position in the mediastinum. This lateral deflection of the lung and pleura due to the heart creates a space that is referred to as the 'cardiac notch'.

The mentioned surface markings of the lungs are according to when they are mid-inspiration.

Good Medical Practice

When identifying T1-T3, find the vertebra prominens (C7) first then palpate down to the vertebra you are looking for.

T3 is also in level with the spine of scapula, so that is an alternative guide to help you identify nearby vertebrae. The surface markings of lobes of the lungs become a lot clearer after you understand the surface markings of the fissures.

3 The surface markings of the fissures of the right and left lungs

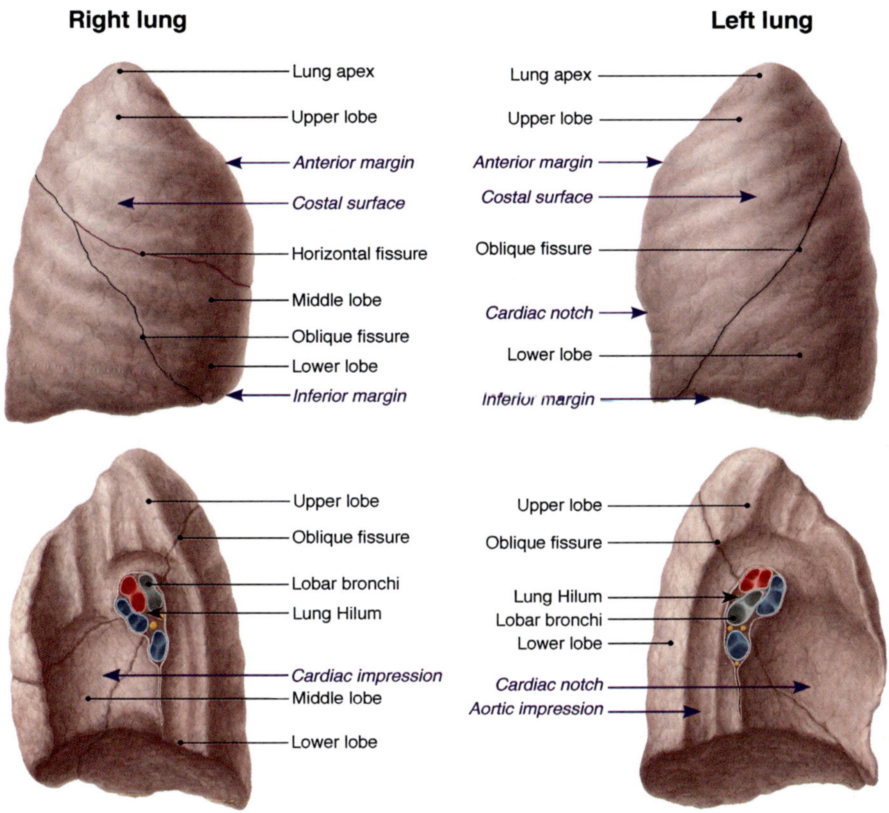

Fig 3.5 Lateral and medial views of the lungs highlighting the fissures which separate the lobes. Pulmonary arteries in the hilum are represented in red and pulmonary veins are represented in blue. However, this is not representative of the oxygen saturation of the blood that flows through them, as pulmonary veins carry oxygenated blood to the left atrium and pulmonary arteries transport deoxygenated blood coming from the right ventricle. The colour coding is designed to help you more easily remember the locations of the vessels in the hilum.

Oblique fissure of right lung	Oblique fissure of left lung
Separates the inferior (lower) lobe of the right lung from the superior (upper) and middle lobes.	Separates the inferior lobe of the left lung from the superior lobe.

Demonstration of the oblique fissure in both lungs:

Ask the patient to sit up and palpate the lung border at level T3 posteriorly, which is in level with the spine of the scapula. On the anterior chest wall, identify the 6th CC, the lower border of the lung. Finally, connect the two points around the lateral thoracic wall.

Transverse (horizontal) fissure of right lung

Separates the superior lobe of the right lung from the middle lobe.

Demonstration of the transverse fissure in the right lung:

Identify the right 4th CC by palpating down from the sternal angle. Draw a line extending along the 4th rib to meet the oblique fissure at the MAL near the axilla (runs above the nipple in males). When demonstrating this on a patient, you do not need to ask the patient to sit up as there are no posterior surface markings.

Good Medical Practice

When identifying T1-T3, find the vertebra prominens (C7) first then palpate down to the vertebra you are looking for. T3 is also in level with the spine of scapula, so that is an alternative guide to help you identify nearby vertebrae.
The surface markings of lobes of the lungs become a lot clearer after you understand the surface markings of the fissures.

Although the learning objective requires description of the surface markings, they can also ask you to demonstrate the fissures and lobes in the exam. So, practice how to demonstrate both, as well as describing them.

4 The surface markings of the inferior and mediastinal margins of the parietal pleura of the right and left lungs

The parietal pleura lines the walls of the thoracic cavity and is closely associated with the diaphragm above the costal margin inferiorly, and the mediastinum medially.[15]

When identifying the surface marking on the MAL, ask the patient to move their hand to the back of their head so you can demonstrate clearly to the examiner.

The mediastinal pleura is a part of the parietal pleura that surrounds the mediastinum. When asked for the surface markings of the mediastinal pleura, identify the parasternal borders, including the cardiac notch.

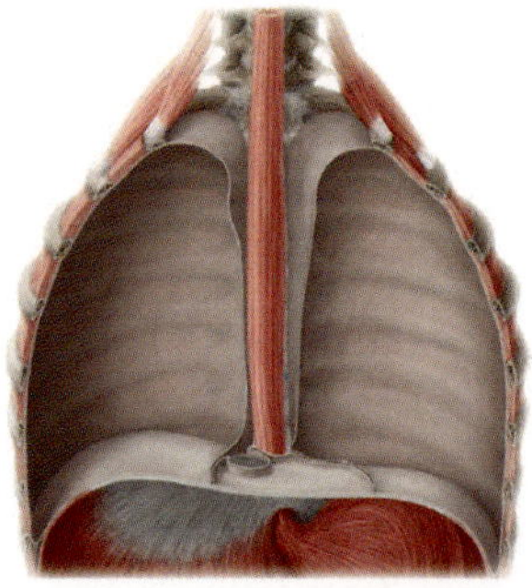

Fig 3.6 The posterior costal margins and inferior borders of the parietal pleura. The coronal illustration depicts a slice posterior to the heart and mediastinum, and so the only parietal pleural margin of significance for this learning objective is the inferior margin.

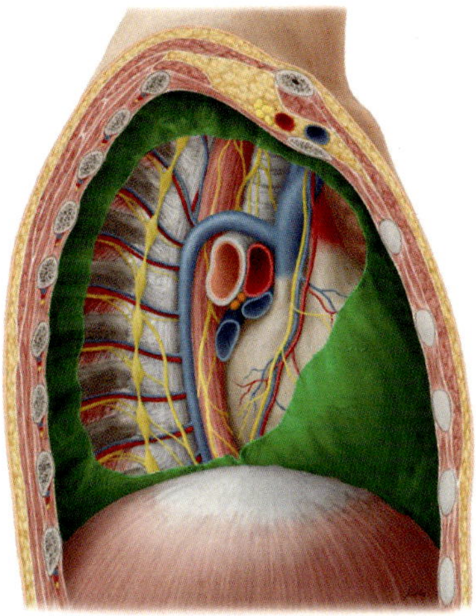

Fig 3.7 Sagittal illustration of the parietal pleura, represented in green.

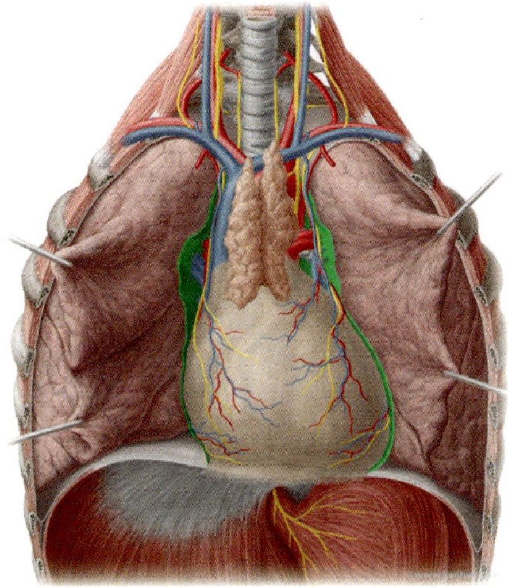

Fig 3.8 The parietal pleura in relation to the other viscera of the thorax. The mediastinal pleura is highlighted in green for ease of viewing.

Surface markings of the parietal pleura on the chest wall

Right parietal pleura	Left parietal pleura
Apex is 2-3cm above medial third of right clavicle	Apex is 2-3cm above medial third of left clavicle
Right sternoclavicular joint	Left sternoclavicular joint
2nd CC at sternal angle	2nd CC at sternal angle
4th CC at sternal border (parasternal line)	*Deflect sharply to the left (2-3cm) compared to the right parietal pleura due to cardiac notch*
6th CC at sternal border (parasternal line)	
8th rib at the MCL	8th rib at the MCL
10th rib at the MAL	10th rib at the MAL
12th Vertebra at the scapular line (posterior chest wall)	12th Vertebra at the scapular line (posterior chest wall)
L1 vertebra transverse process at PML	L1 vertebra transverse process at PML

5 The surface markings of the visceral pleural margins of the right and left lungs

The visceral pleura adheres to the lungs; hence its inferior borders are more superior to the parietal pleura, and closely follow the borders of the lungs. Therefore, when you are describing the borders of the visceral pleura, you are also describing the borders of the lung in question.

Furthermore, the margins of the visceral pleura and the parietal pleura are very closely associated until the 6th costal cartilage at the parasternal line. Although, from this point, the parietal pleural margins continue inferiorly relative to the visceral pleura, leaving a distance of 2 ribs.

Right visceral pleura	Left visceral pleura
Apex is 2-3cm above medial third of right clavicle	Apex is 2-3cm above medial third of left clavicle
Right sternoclavicular joint	Left sternoclavicular joint
2nd CC at sternal angle	2nd CC at sternal angle
4th CC at sternal border (parasternal line)	*Deflect sharply to the left (2-3cm) compared to the right visceral pleura due to cardiac notch*
6th CC at sternal border (parasternal line)	
6th rib at the MCL	6th rib at the MCL
8th rib at the MAL	8th rib at the MAL
10th Vertebra at the scapular line (posterior chest wall)	10th Vertebra at the scapular line (posterior chest wall)

Learning notes

The visceral and parietal pleura are continuous with each other, and they are formed of a single layer of mesothelium and a supporting connective tissue. The lungs do not completely fill up the regions of pleural cavities, resulting in recesses. This is where fluids can be collected and aspirated upon.[15]

6 Investigation for symmetrical lung inflation

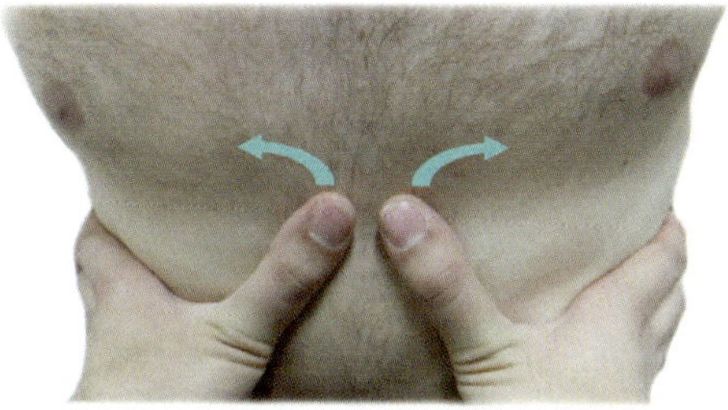

Fig 3.9 Investigation for symmetrical lung inflation performed anteriorly.

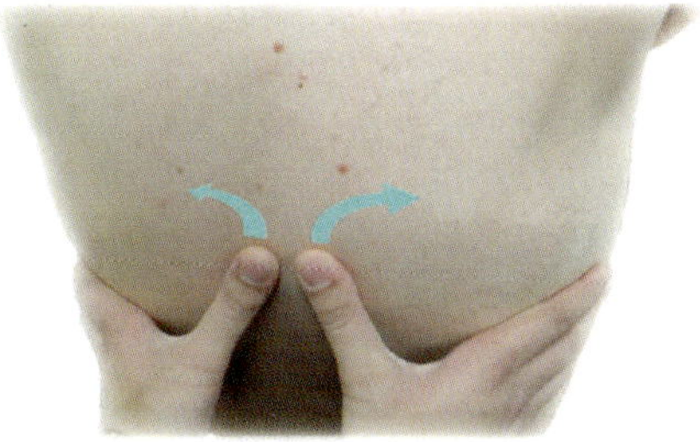

Fig 3.10 Investigation for symmetrical lung inflation performed posteriorly.

Procedure:

1) Gain consent to touch the patient's chest for examining their breathing.
"*Would it be alright if I held my hands around your chest to check your breathing?*"
2) Place your hands around the lateral ribcage, as shown in **Fig. 3.7**, pulling forward the skin from behind the MAL without stabilizing your thumbs on to the patient yet.
3) Ask the patient to exhale, and stretch your thumbs towards the midline so that they lightly touch. This is so that the thumb moves apart easily when the patient breathes in and out.
4) Then ask the patient to take a deep breath in, measure by eye how much the thumbs move apart in each direction, and out, the thumbs should come back to its original place.
5) Repeat this for another breath in and out and remember to hold your thumb loosely but the rest of the fingers tightly.
6) Observations: thumbs move apart at an equal distance of 2-3cm in each direction, indicating normal chest expansion.
7) Report back to the examiner what you have observed.
"*The lungs are expanding symmetrically, as my thumbs moved apart equally in each direction by about 2-3cm.*"

Medical notes

Chest expansion can be decreased by lung disease such as pneumonia or collapsed lung; unilateral decrease could be due to a pleural effusion and bilateral decrease could be due to diseases such as chronic obstructive pulmonary diseases (COPD).[16]

7 Investigate the breathing pattern and breathing rate of a patient

Procedure:

1) Whilst the patient is lying down on the bed, relaxed, inform them that you will be taking some measurements. It is completely fine in the OSPEs to tell the patient that you will be recording their breathing rate, but just remember that patients knowing that you are looking at their breathing may influence their resting respiratory rate, so doctors may often take the respiratory rate whilst they pretend to take their pulse.
   "*I am going to have a look at your breathing, is that okay with you?*"

2) Count the number of breaths the patient takes in 30 seconds, and multiply this by 2 when reporting the number of breaths per minute to the examiner.

3) Report back to the examiner your findings.
   "*This patient has a respiratory rate of n breaths per minute, which is normal/low/high. Breathing pattern was regular/irregular.*"

   * Make sure that when you are reporting back to the examiner, the respiratory rate you give is a multiple of 2. As the OSPE recruits normal people as 'patients', the respiratory rate and pattern will almost always be normal and regular.

Medical notes

Abnormal breathing patterns can be picked up by just this simple investigation through inspection. The usual respiratory rate for adults is 12-16 breaths per minute. Some different breathing patterns may suggest specific disorders:

Rapid shallow breathing – hyperventilation episodes, interstitial lung disease

Prolonged expiratory phase – significant airway obstruction e.g. asthma or COPD

Kussmaul's respiration – rapid deep sighing breathing pattern, aka 'air hunger', caused by acidosis e.g. diabetic ketoacidosis.[16]

8 Percussion of the lobes of the left and right lungs

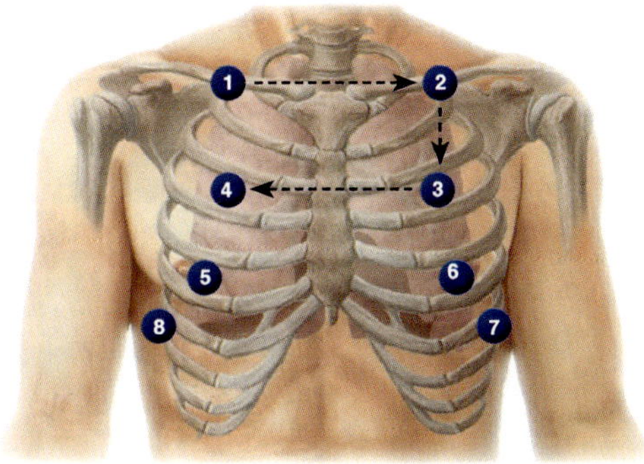

Fig 3.11 Anterior chest wall with markings of suggested percussion sites.

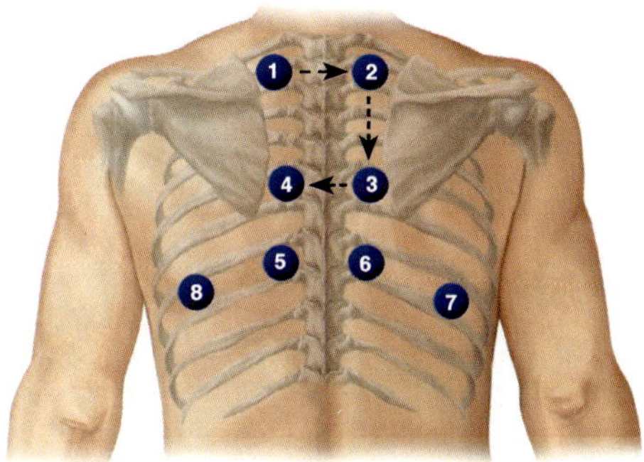

Fig 3.12 Posterior chest wall with markings of suggested percussion sites.

Chest percussion technique:[17]

1) Obtain the patient's consent before you begin percussion.
   "I will now tap down on your chest."

2) Press the distal and middle phalanges of your non-dominant finger (usually middle finger) firmly and directly on an intercostal space and raise the second and fourth fingers off the chest surface.

3) With a quick motion of the wrist, tap onto the finger 2 times on the chest wall with the tip of a finger (usually middle finger) of the other hand. The best percussion site is between the proximal and distal interphalangeal joints.

* The exception to this rule is when you are percussing the clavicle – where there should be no underlying finger and percussed directly on to the bone.
I highly recommend watching videos to ensure you are getting the right sound and technique, along with frequently practicing on yourself and your peers.

	Anterior Chest Wall:	*Posterior Chest Wall:*
Upper lobe	1) Medial 1/3rd of clavicle (directly onto bone) 2) Any point on the anterior chest wall infraclavicular and above 4th rib for right lung, above 5th rib for left lung (e.g. 3rd ICS at MCL)	1) At level T1 and T3 between the scapular line and the vertebral column

Middle lobe of right lung

Anterior Chest Wall:

1) 4th or 5th ICS (just under the nipple for men)
2) Just below the axilla at MAL

Lower lobe

Anterior Chest Wall:	*Posterior Chest Wall:*
1) 6th or 7th ICS near MAL (just under the base of the breast in females)	1) Anywhere between the scapula to T10 (e.g. 8th rib at scapular line)

Do not forget to percuss posteriorly, especially for the lower lobes. Before you proceed to percuss on the back, ask the patient to sit up with their feet over the edge of the bed. You should also ask them to cross their arms (like they are hugging themselves) so that the scapula is pulled out of the way.

It is always useful to develop your own system of going through the percussion sites. The suggested way is going superior to inferior, moving across to the symmetrical site on the other lung, right to left.

It is not necessary to palpate for each anatomical location to percuss as long as you are percussing within the borders of the lobe asked by the examiner.

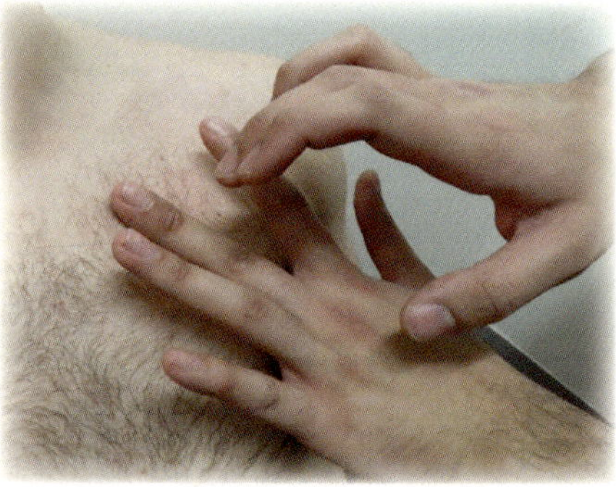

Fig 3.13 Percussion of a patients thorax.

Medical notes

Percussion determines if parts of the thoracic cavity are filled with foreign subjects. When the percussion note resonates like a drum, it indicates that the lung is air filled which you would find in a normal lung. A dull sound is produced in the presence of fluid or when tissue density is increased, a flat sound suggests there is solid in the pleural space and a hyperresonant sound is heard in the case of pneumothorax.[16,17]

9 Auscultation of the lobes of the left and right lungs

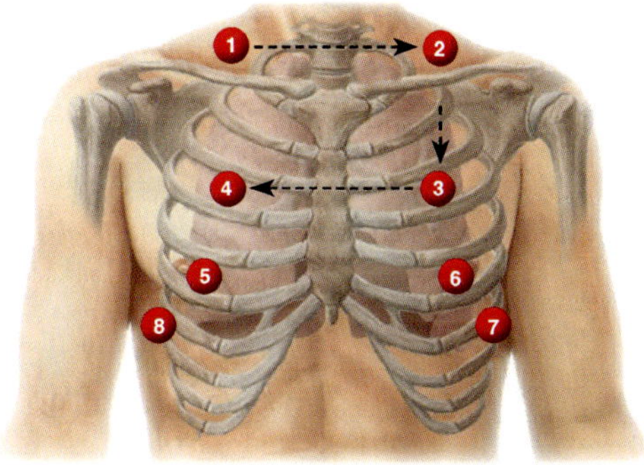

Fig 3.14 Anterior chest wall with markings of suggested auscultation sites.

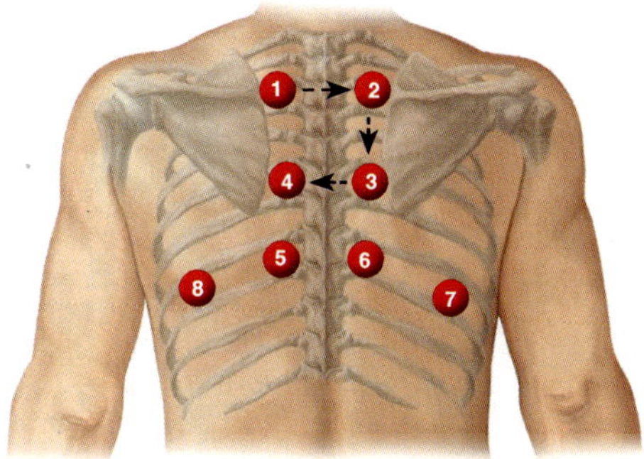

Fig 3.15 Posterior chest wall with markings of suggested auscultation sites.

Chest auscultation technique:

1) Obtain the patient's consent before you begin percussion, and tell them that you will be listening to their breathing.
   "*I will now have a listen to your chest through the stethoscope. It might feel a little cold.*"
2) Place the earpieces in your ears so that they are pointing antero-medially (pointing into your ear canal).
3) Ensure the diaphragm is engaged by lightly tapping onto it. If not, twist the head of the stethoscope.
4) Place the stethoscope on the patient firmly and ask them to take a deep breath in and out every time you move the stethoscope's position to auscultate.

	Anterior Chest Wall:	*Posterior Chest Wall:*
Upper lobe	1) Lung apex (just above the medial third of clavicle) 2) Any point on the anterior chest wall infraclavicular and above 4th rib for right lung, above 5th rib for left lung (e.g. 3rd ICS at MCL)	1) Upper back near scapula spine (level T3)

Middle lobe of right lung

Anterior Chest Wall:
1) 5th ICS at MCL (just under the nipple for men) 2) Just below the axilla at MAL

Lower lobe	Anterior Chest Wall:	Posterior Chest Wall:
	1) 6th or 7th ICS near MAL (just under the base of the breast in females)	1) Anywhere between the scapula to T10 (e.g. 8th rib at scapular line)

When auscultating the apex, use the bell of the stethoscope. For the rest of the auscultation, use the diaphragm.

For auscultation on the back, ask the patient to sit up with their feet over the edge of the bed before you proceed, with their arms in a position such that they are hugging themselves.

Observations: In a healthy individual, a sound should be heard during inspiration, with less noise produced on expiration.

As with percussion, compare the sounds at symmetrical points on each side before progressing to the next point of the chest.

Good Medical Practice

The bell filters out high-frequency sounds so it is appropriate for listening to low-frequency sounds, known as vesicular sounds. The diaphragm, on the other hand, detects high-frequency sounds, known as bronchial sounds. Breathing sounds from the chest are normally high-pitched, hence the diaphragm is used for most of the auscultation.

Intensity of sound is a function of airflow. Diminished or absent breath sounds may have been caused by airway obstruction, hyperinflation, pneumothorax, pleural effusion or obesity.

In obstructive airway diseases, such as asthma, there may be normal breath sounds but with prolonged expiration. There can also be wheezes, commonly caused by asthma and COPD, or crackles, due to pneumonia or bronchiectasis.[18,19]

10 Describe and demonstrate the triangle of safety for a chest drain

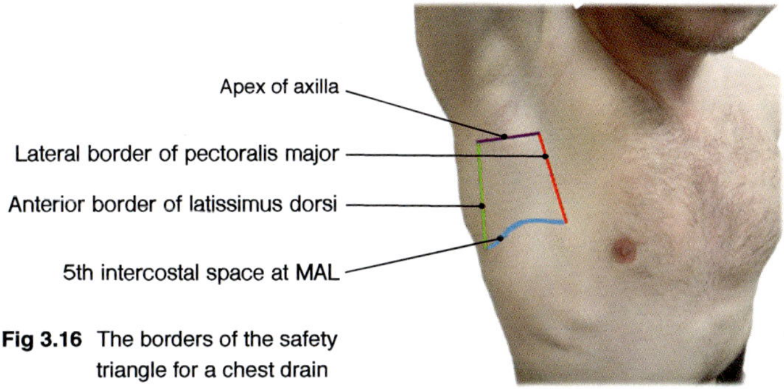

Fig 3.16 The borders of the safety triangle for a chest drain

Before demonstration, ask the patient to move the hand on the side you are going to demonstrate to the back of their head, so they are lying on their hand.

Borders of the safety triangle

Posterior	Anterior border of latissimus dorsi (posterior axillary fold)
Anterior	Lateral border of pectoralis major (anterior axillary fold)
Inferior	5th intercostal space at MAL
Superior	Below apex of axilla

The triangle of safety overlies 2nd to 5th intercostal spaces. To show this, you can palpate along from the sternal angle (2nd CC).

When asked to describe, make sure you are not demonstrating:
"The posterior border for the safety triangle is the anterior border of latissimus dorsi, the anterior border is the lateral border of pectoralis major, the inferior border is the 5th intercostal space at the mid-axillary line and the superior border is at the base of the apex of the axilla."

You may be asked to describe and demonstrate, in which case point and act out the borders on the patient as you talk through each border.

Medical Notes

Chest drains are indicated in certain lung conditions such as pneumothorax, pleural effusion, haemothorax or post-operative lungs.[20] This triangle of safety shows the area on the lateral chest wall where it is possible to insert a chest drain without damaging any nearby nerves such as the long thoracic nerve.

Final Remarks

As you can see, the respiratory station is heavily based on the surface anatomy of the lungs, and once you master that the rest should follow.

When you are asked to describe and demonstrate or just demonstrate, demonstrate directly on the patient and describe what you are doing at the same time. For example, if you are finding the 4th rib by palpating 2 ribs down from the sternal angle, explain that you are doing exactly so!

If the examiner asks something that you were not prepared to do, you can ask the examiner to repeat the question to clarify what you are required to do and prepare for what you can answer – even if it is a part of the question. Do not be afraid of stating that you do not have the answer when you don't. When you have time at the end of the station, you can go back to the question that you missed so don't let a single question trip your whole station up.

When practicing with your friends, give thorough feedback to each other and learn from your mistakes to avoid repeating them. Like it says on the tin, this is a practical exam, so saying and acting out everything and using another person to help you is the best way of revision.

Good luck! Hope you all ace your exams.

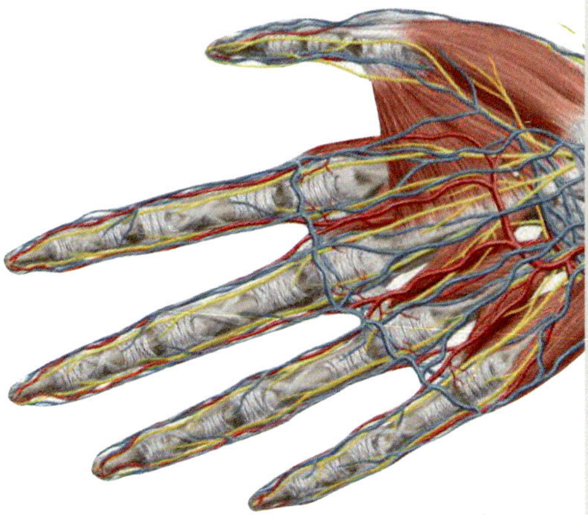

The Cardiovascular System

By Arian Arjomandi Rad

Introduction to the chapter

The following chapter will help you acquire a solid knowledge of the surface anatomy and clinical skills of the cardiovascular system. The knowledge acquired for this station will not only be essential to pass the OSPE station but will also ensure that you have an understanding of what is arguably one of the most important systems in terms of pathology and physiology in our body.

Cardiovascular disease affects and poses a threat to the lives of millions of people around the world, with Coronary Artery Disease (CAD) classifying itself as the number one killer in the U.K.[21]
This means that it is imperative for you, as a medical student, to be familiar and know the basics of the system, which will form the key foundations to your clinical years. Indeed, being able to firstly correctly identify what is physiological from the pathological could be considered one of the most important steps in your learning.

In comparison to the other OSPE stations, the cardiovascular one has the least number of Learning Outcomes. Furthermore, the level of difficulty of the tasks you will be required to perform will be lower than the ones of other stations. However, this deems the station or the knowledge covered no less important than any other station; in fact, this means that it becomes harder for polished clinical skills to stand out.

This chapter will cover all the L.O.s providing you with the knowledge needed to outstand in the exam. A section of Good Medical practice and author's tip will be also provided for each LO.

Clinical Communication

"I have been asked to perform a chest examination on you, and this involves me having a feel of different parts of your chest and listening to your heart using my stethoscope. Is that ok with you?"

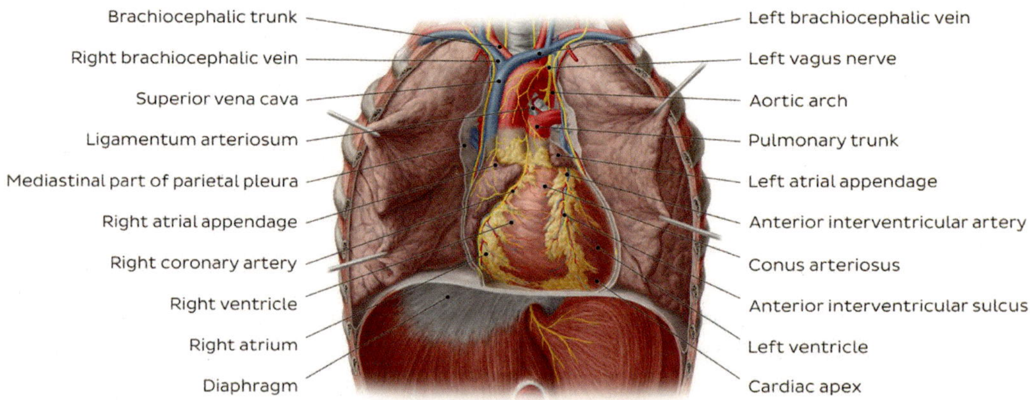

Fig 4.1 The heart in situ.

1 The surface markings of the borders of the heart

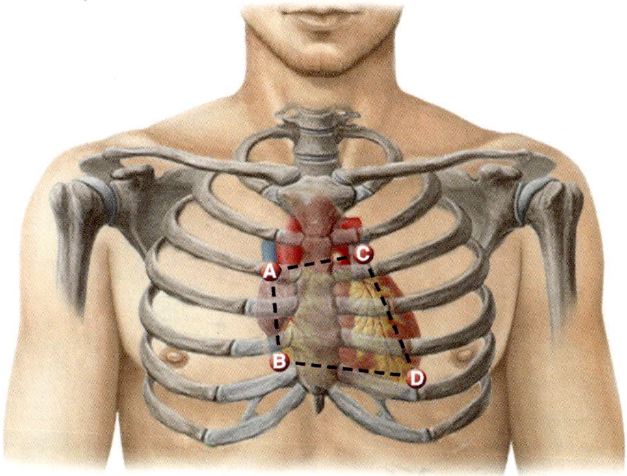

Fig 4.2 The surface anatomy of the borders of the heart.

To demonstrate the borders of the heart on a patient; you should essentially connect the four highlighted points on the diagram above.

- **Right Border:**
  From the 3rd right costal cartilage, 1cm lateral to the sternal border (**A**), to the 6th right costal cartilage (**B**).

- **Left Border:**
  From the 2nd left intercostal space (ICS), 2.5cm from the sternal border (**C**), to the 5th intercostal space at the midclavicular line (**D**).

- **Upper border:**
  From the 3rd right costal cartilage, 1cm lateral to the sternum (**A**), to the 2nd left intercostal space, 2.5cm from the sternal border (**C**).

- **Lower border:**
  From the 6th right costal cartilage (**B**) to the 5th intercostal space at midclavicular line (**D**).

You will have to demonstrate the borders to the examiner by explaining their location and physically highlighting the borders your fingers.

Good Medical Practice

First of all, make sure you are confident with the anatomical position (including the left and right side of a patient). It is not unusual for students to confuse the left and right side on a patient during demonstrations in the OSPE stations, which immediately highlights the candidate as amateur and unprepared to the examiner.

Always remember that the apex of the heart sits on the left 5th ICS at the mid-clavicular line.[22] It is possible to check if the areas you have defined are correct by percussing the heart for dullness. An expanded area of dullness (e.g. to the mid-axillary line) is suggestive of cardiomegaly or pericardial effusion.[23]

Also, whenever locating any ICS or costal cartilage, you should start counting from the second ICS found laterally to the sternal angle of Louis, at the level of T4/5.

Mastering the surface anatomy is crucial to the clinical assessment interpretation of radiological findings, and particularly for thoracic surgery incision. Understanding both the surface and the deeper anatomy of the heart will be imperative in the placement of Electrocardiogram (ECG) leads and in avoiding lead misplacement.[24]

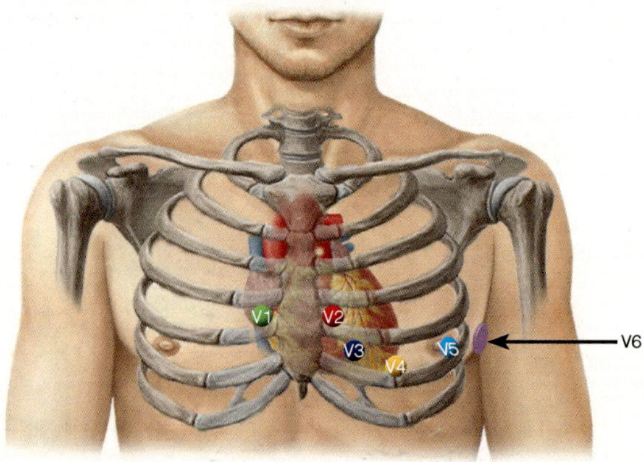

Fig 4.3 Placement of the ECG chest leads.

V1: Right 4th ICS next to the sternum.
V2: Left 4th ICS next to the sternum.
V3: Left 5th ICS between V2 & V4.
V4: Left 5th ICS at mid-clavicular line.
V5: Left 5th ICS at anterior-axillary line.
V6: Left 5th ICS at mid-axillary line

2 Auscultation of the heart valves

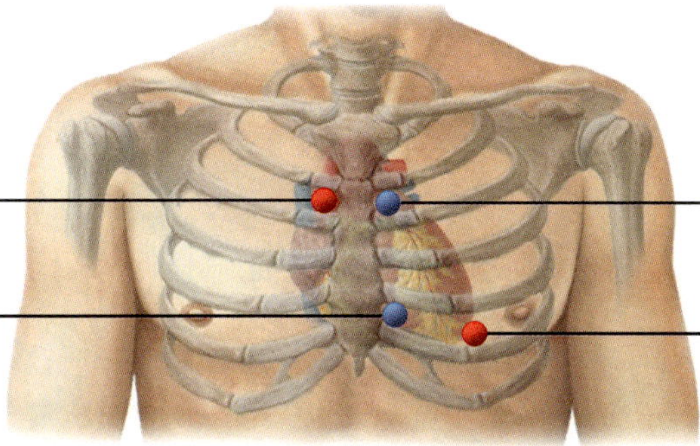

Fig 4.4 Anatomical locations for the auscultation of the heart valves. Red markers represent the locations of the valves in the systemic circulatory system, and blue markers represent valves in the pulmonary circulatory system.

The anatomical positions where you would auscultate for the valves are as follows:[22,23]

Auscultation of the **aortic** valve is at the RIGHT 2nd ICS at the sternal border.
Auscultation of the **pulmonary** valve is at the LEFT 2nd ICS at the sternal border.
Auscultation of the **tricuspid** valve is at the LEFT 5th ICS at the sternal border.
Auscultation of the **mitral** valve is at the LEFT 5th ICS at the mid-clavicular line, at the location of the apex beat.

Use the diaphragm of the stethoscope (for high-pitch sounds) to listen to the aortic, pulmonary, and tricuspid valves. For the mitral valve, begin by using the bell of the stethoscope (for low pitched sounds), and then switch to the diaphragm.
Also, auscultate for the valves in that order: aortic → pulmonary → tricuspid → mitral.

Vital OSPE Knowledge

To listen for valve sounds, you should position your stethoscope downstream from the flow of blood through the valves. This means that the sites of auscultation of the heart valves differ from their anatomical location, although you are required to know both locations.

The anatomical locations of the four heart valves are as follows:

The **aortic** valve is obliquely-aligned at the RIGHT 3rd ICS at the sternal border.
The **pulmonary** valve is horizontal and located at the LEFT 3rd costal cartilage.
The **tricuspid** valve is vertical and at the RIGHT 4th ICS at the sternal border.
The **mitral** valve is oblique and at the LEFT 4th ICS at the sternal border.

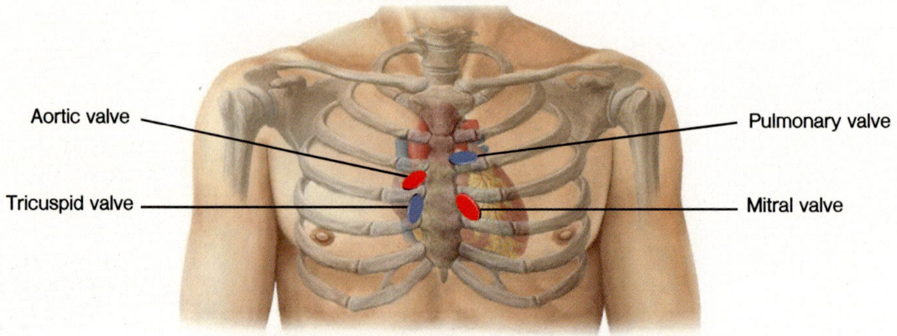

Fig 4.5 Anatomical locations of the heart valves.

The tricuspid is auscultated on the left side but is anatomically on the right side, and all the valves on the right side are found at ICS while on the left are at costal cartilages. Remember, you cannot auscultate at costal cartilages. This might help you remember the actual anatomical locations better.

Good Medical Practice

Remember, palpate for the sternal angle (of Louis) to easily locate the second intercostal space before you place your stethoscope anywhere on the patient's body. It's also good practice to touch the diaphragm of your stethoscope before using it, to make sure it's not cold enough to cause significant discomfort to the patient. Also, as mentioned in the previous learning objectives, don't forget to follow the etiquettes of palpation when performing this task.
Also, you use the bell of the diaphragm first when auscultating the mitral valve to listen out for mitral stenosis.

Extra Medical Knowledge

The first heart sound (S1), known as the "lub", occurs at the beginning of systole and is the result of the closure of the two atrioventricular valves (mitral and tricuspid).[23] The second heart sound (S2), known as the "dub", occurs at the end of systole and it results from the closure of the aortic and pulmonary valves. Both sounds are caused by turbulence when the blood is flowing through the valves as the valves are closing.[25] The auscultatory findings can also be related to the cardiac cycle by palpating the carotid artery while auscultating the valves. S1 precedes the carotid pulse while S2 follows the carotid pulse.[26]

Also, two other heart sounds (S3 and S4), known as gallops, may be present both physiologically and pathologically, although this is beyond the scope of the OSPE. The best way to listen to these sounds is by lightly using the bell of the stethoscope.[27] The presence of S3 in old people could indicate congestive heart failure while in younger people, especially athletes, might be a physiological finding.[28] S4 takes place at the end of diastole and might be indicative of coronary artery disease or left ventricular hypertrophy (which can be caused by hypertension). To distinguish between S3 and S4, remember that S3 has the cadence of the word "Kentucky", while the S4 has the cadence of "Tennesee".[29] Look this up! Note that in case of atrial fibrillation the fourth sound will not be heard due to inefficient atrial contraction.

3 Examination of the radial, ulnar, brachial, and carotid pulse, and subsequent findings

To examine the radial, ulnar, two brachial, and carotid pulses you will have to be confident with their anatomical landmark.

After finding the anatomical landmarks (described below), place the pads of your index and middle finger (do not use your thumb) on the landmark and lightly palpate the wall of the artery. Make sure you do not press too hard as you might obliterate the pulse, thus not being able to feel anything.

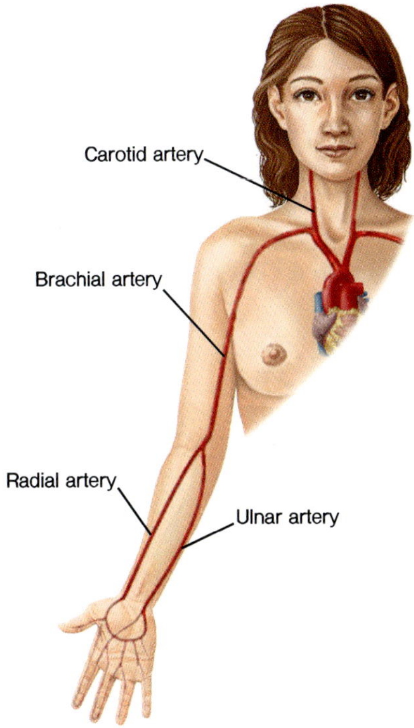

Fig 4.6 The key arteries of pulse taking in the upper limb and neck.

Carotid artery:

The carotid pulse arises from the common carotid artery and can be found at the anterior border of the SCM at the level of the superior border of the laryngeal prominence (Adam's apple).

Expose the neck of the patient. Place your index and middle finger pads at the anterior triangle of the neck anteriorly to the sternocleidomastoid muscle and lateral to the larynx (simply, halfway in between the two). Don't occlude the artery for too long, and certainly don't take the pulse from both carotid arteries at the same time.

Once you found the pulse at any location, take the pulse rate of the patient for 30s as is required in the OSPE, and multiply it by two to obtain the beats per minute (bpm). Make sure you state to the examiner that you would ideally take the pulse for one full minute, but due to time constraints, you are only taking it for 30s and multiplying it.

Please avoid taking the carotid pulse on both sides simultaneously, as occlusion of both carotid arteries at the same time can result in the patient fainting, which will not result well in the OSPEs.

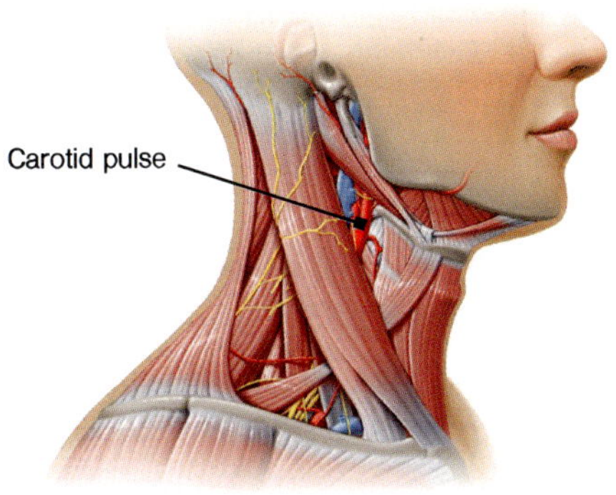

Fig 4.7 The location to palpate for the carotid pulse.

Good Medical Practice

To see the anterior border of the SCM, ask the patient to look to one side. Then place your finder at the anterior border of the SCM at the level of the laryngeal prominence and ask the patient to face forward again. Only take the pulse when the patient faces forward since the medial head of the SCM will cover the pulse when the patient is looking to the side. Pulses are best felt by pushing against a bony structure, and in this case, directly posterior onto the transverse process of the adjacent cervical vertebra.

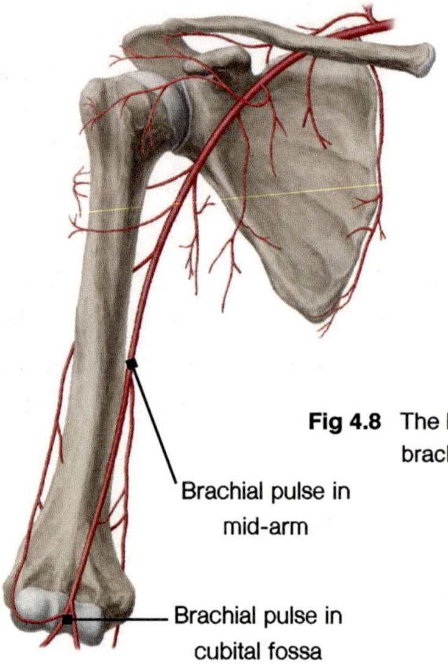

Fig 4.8 The locations to palpate for the brachial pulse in the arm.

Brachial artery:

There are two sites where the brachial pulse could be felt.

The first one is in the mid-arm:
On the medial side of the arm between the biceps brachii and the triceps brachii tendon.

The second one is at the cubital fossa:
The brachial artery is positioned medial the biceps bacchii muscles tendon. Make sure that the arm is relaxed when examining to avoid the muscles from covering the artery.

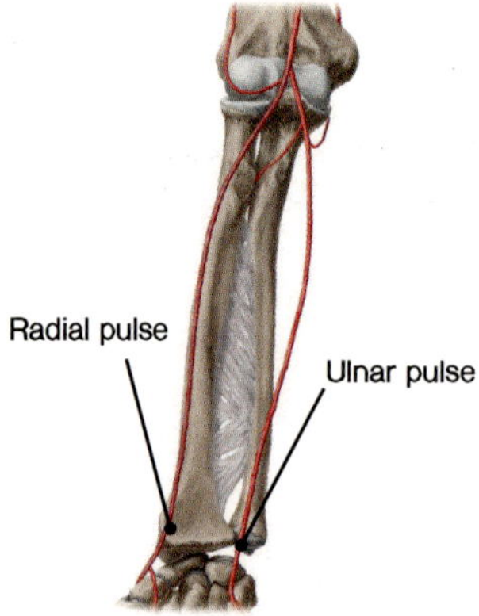

Fig 4.9 The locations to palpate for the radial and ulnar pulse in the forearm.

Radial artery:

Expose the patient's wrist with the palm open and facing upwards. Position your index and middle finger on the radial side of the wrist (around 2cm below the base of the thumb). The radial artery is located lateral to the tendon of the flexor carpi radialis muscle, and you will be pressing the radial artery on the radial bone to palpate for a pulse.

Ulnar artery:

Expose the patient's wrist with the palm open and facing upwards. Position your index and middle finger on the ulnar side of the wrist. The ulnar artery is located proximal to the pisiform and under the lateral border of the flexor carpi ulnaris tendon, and you will be pressing the ulnar artery on the head of the ulna to palpate for a pulse.

Pulse rate:

Remember that the normal resting heart rate of a person is between 60 and 100 bpm.
Also, remember that the examiner will check the pulse of the patient at the same time as you, so do not make the number up.

Rhythm:

Since OSPE is a pre-clinical exam, you simply have to note whether the pulse has a normal (sinus) rhythm or is irregular.

Good Medical Practice

Finding the pulse of a person might not always be an easy task, especially if the patient's pulse is rather weak. In such a scenario, it is easy to stress out/panic during the exam and you might be tempted to make the number up. You should avoid this as the examiner will be taking the pulse with you at the same time, albeit not at the same contralateral position.

Also, the examiner will not accept "I cannot find the pulse of the patient because it's weak" as a valid excuse. The best thing to do is to take your time (i.e. a couple of seconds more) and try to find the pulse! Keep practicing this examination aspect with as many different people as you can.

Pulse rate: tachycardia is defined as a pulse rate of over 100bpm while bradycardia is defined as a rate of below 60bpm.[30] Bradycardia is not always pathological and might be present in athletes.

4 Palpate the apex beat of the heart

For the purposes of this exam, you should know that the apex beat of the heart is located, and can be palpated, at the left 5th ICS at the mid-clavicular line.

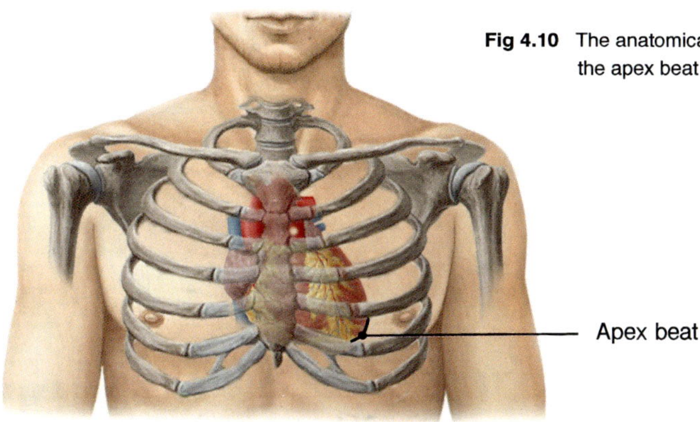

Fig 4.10 The anatomical location of the apex beat of the heart.

With the patient's thorax exposed, and the patient lying on the bed positioned at a 45° angle, the procedure is as follows:

- From the sternal angle of Louis, work your way down to the 5th ICS. Make sure you count down the ribs and do not just jump the to the apex beat.
- Once at the 5th intercostal space start more laterally and move medially towards the midclavicular line. This to eliminate the possibility of a laterally deviated apex beat as a result of cardiomegaly.[31]
- Palpate by having the palm of your hand on the patient and using the middle three fingers. The middle finger should go at the intercostal space while the other two fingers should be on the ribs above and below the ICS.

Good Medical Practice

In certain cases, the apex beat is not always at the 5th ICS at the midclavicular line. For example, in children the apex beat is located at the 4th ICS,[32] and in cardiomegaly, the apex beat can deviate laterally to the mid-axillary line.

Furthermore, when palpating the apex beat, several aspects including the location, amplitude, size, presence of thrills, and duration of the beat should be considered.
In fact, the presence of the apex beat is the first thing you should consider. Indeed, the absence of the apex beat could have several physiological and pathological causes.

A good mnemonic for the causes of the absence is DR POPE:

Physiological:
D – Dextrocardia (a rare condition in which the heart points towards the right side of the chest)
R – Ribs (should the apex beat be behind a rib, lie the patient down on their left side and repeat)

Pathological:
P – Pericardial effusion (abnormal accumulation of fluid around the heart in the pericardial sac)
O – Obesity
P – Pleural effusion (abnormal accumulation of fluid in the pleura)
E – Emphysema (significant breakdown of the alveoli)

Also, a quicker, yet much less accurate method exists in locating the 5th ICS. This is by knowing that the male nipple is located at the 4th ICS and working down from there. However, in females, the location of the nipple can vary significantly respective of the breast size. Although, it is widely taught that the female breast is usually from the 2nd to the 6th rib.[33]

Furthermore, the comfort of the patient must be considered when palpating for the apex beat. With female patients, ask them to lift their breast should it be obstructing the apex beat palpation.

5 Routine venepuncture sites

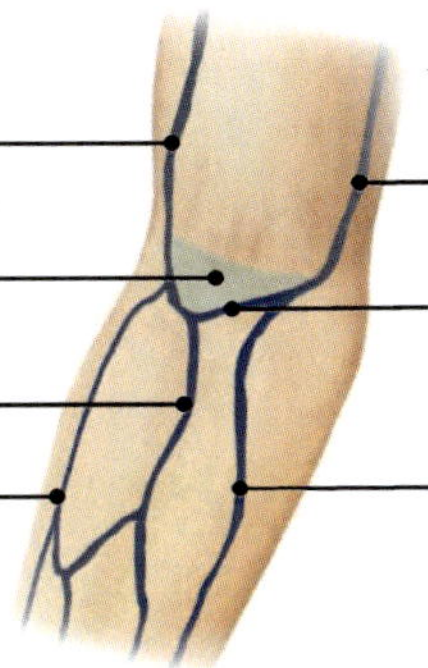

Fig 4.11 The prominent superficial veins of the arm and forearm, along with the depression known as the cubital fossa.

For this LO, you are required to describe and identify the antebrachial vein, the median cubital vein, and the cubital fossa. Remember, because it is a learning objective which requires you to demonstrate, you must be able to physically point out the appropriate veins on the patient.

When required to point out the most common site of venepuncture you should start by showing the examiner the borders of the cubital fossa: Brachioradialis muscle (medial border), the pronator teres muscle (lateral border), and an imaginary line between the two epicondyles of the humerus (superior border).

Once you have located the borders of the cubital fossa, identify the biceps brachii tendon. The median cubital vein, which is an anastomosis of the cephalic and basilic veins, is located medially to the tendon.

Note: It might be helpful to know the contents of the cubital fossa (laterally to medially): **radial nerve**, **biceps brachii tendon**, **median cubital vein**, **brachial artery**, **median nerve**.

Good Medical Practice

To physically point out the antebrachial or median cubital veins on the patient at the station, you will likely have to make them more prominent. To do this, you should ask the patient to repeatedly make fists while you constrict their arm using two hands (one hand on the anterior arm, and the other hand on the posterior arm), as you are not provided with a tourniquet.

Also, it is somewhat easier to identify the medial cubital vein (which is a superficial vein connecting the two prominent veins of the arm and forearm - the basilic and cephalic veins) than it is to identify the antebrachial vein.

Alternative sites to take blood from can be the cephalic vein and the basilic vein, which should be used as last resort due to its higher risk of haematoma. In addition, the dorsal metacarpal veins are another alternative. However, the recommended guidelines for which veins to use as an alternative first vary between healthcare trusts.

6 The surface markings of the aortic arch

The thoracic aorta is composed of three parts: the ascending aorta (coming out of the heart), the aortic arch, and the descending aorta (which becomes the abdominal aorta).
For each of these parts, there is a corresponding surface landmark. However, for the purposes of this exam you will only be required to know the surface markings of the aortic arch, and the other surface markings will be provided as extra knowledge below.

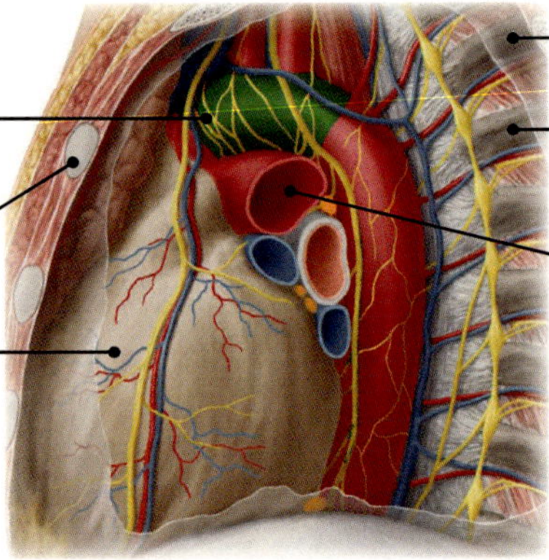

Fig 4.12 Sagittal view of the aortic arch, found behind the manubrium, which has been highlighted in green for ease of viewing.

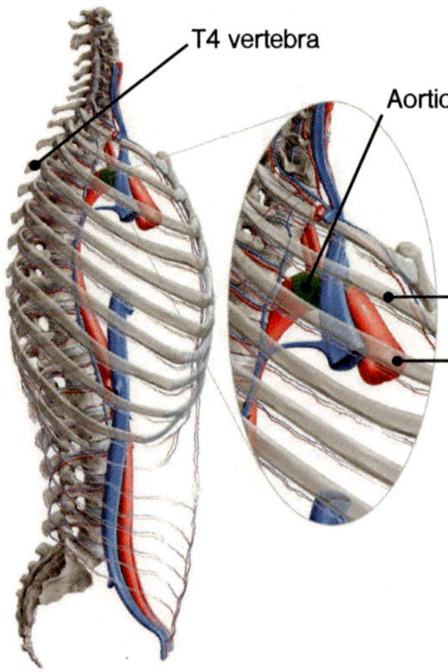

Fig 4.13 The aortic arch relative to the bones of the trunk wall. Again, the aortic arch has been highlighted in green for ease of viewing.

Extra Medical Knowledge

It is common for OSPE examiners to delve deeper into easier LOs such as this by asking extra questions. To ensure full preparedness, it is recommended that you learn the branches that lead off the aortic arch.

From right to left, they arise as: brachiocephalic trunk (which subsequently divides into the right common carotid and subclavian arteries), left common carotid artery, left subclavian artery.

The ascending aorta begins at the lower border of the 3rd costal cartilage and joins the aortic arch at the 2nd costal cartilage.[22]

The descending aorta begins at the 2nd costal cartilage, passing down and medially and ending 2.5cm superior to the transpyloric plane.[22]

7 The surface markings of the internal jugular vein and common carotid artery.

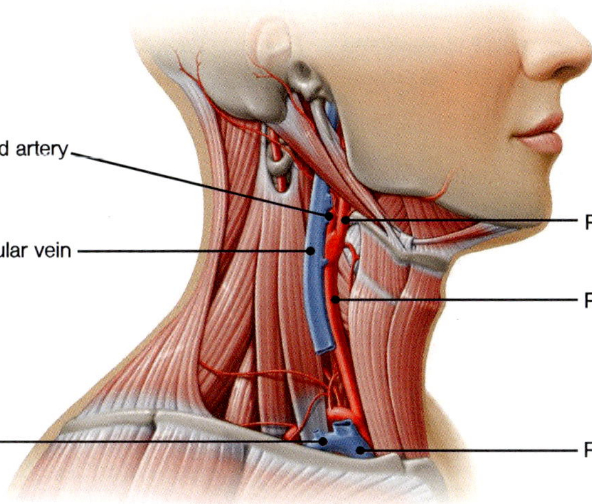

Fig 4.14 The major veins and arteries of the anterior triangle in situ.

For the purpose of this LO, you will be required to know about both the left and right jugular vein and carotid artery. You should be able to point out their position and describe it to the examiner.

The right common carotid artery arises from the brachiocephalic trunk and is situated under the right sternocleidomastoid muscle.
To demonstrate the surface markings, ask the patient to turn their head to the left in order for the right sternocleidomastoid muscle to become clearly prominent. Then, along the anterior muscle border, direct an imaginary line from the right sternoclavicular joint to the right earlobe.

The left common carotid artery arises from the aortic arch and is situated under the left sternocleidomastoid muscle.
To demonstrate the surface markings, ask the patient to turn their head to the right in order for the left sternocleidomastoid muscle to become clearly prominent. Then, along the anterior muscle border, direct an imaginary line from the sternal angle to the left earlobe.

For the left and right internal jugular veins, draw an imaginary line from the respective sternoclavicular joint to the respective earlobe. They run just lateral to the respective carotid arteries.

Extra Medical Knowledge

Although not strictly required for the OSPE examination, knowledge regarding the other main vessels situated in the upper thorax and neck region is vital in clinical education and practice.

The brachiocephalic trunk surface anatomy can be marked by a virtual line connecting the aortic arch to the right sternoclavicular joint. At the right sternoclavicular joint the trunk will bifurcate into the right subclavian and right common carotid artery.

The right and left subclavian arteries can be marked by an arched line from the respective sternoclavicular joint to the midclavicular line at the level of the first rib. You can feel the subclavian artery pulse in the supraclavicular fossa.

The superior vena cava can be marked by a superiorly-pointed virtual line passing behind the right border of the manubrium and sternum, from the 3rd right costal cartilage to the 1st right costal cartilage. Note that the left and right brachiocephalic veins join to form the superior vena cava directly posterior to the right 1st costal cartilage.

8 Describe and demonstrate, on an anatomical model, the main coronary arteries of the heart

Proficiency and knowledge in this most basic of anatomical learning objectives is something which notably lacks amongst pre-clinical medical students. This becomes evident when students enter their clinical years and begin their learning of ECG readings.
Also, this learning objective is created on the examination experiences of past cohort more so than the core skill list.

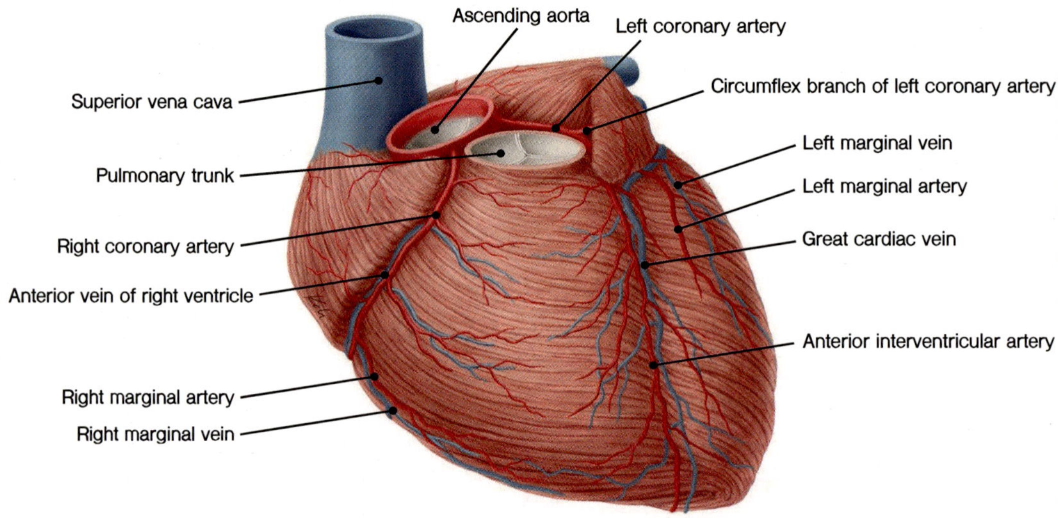

Fig 4.15 The major veins and arteries located on the anterior aspect of the heart.

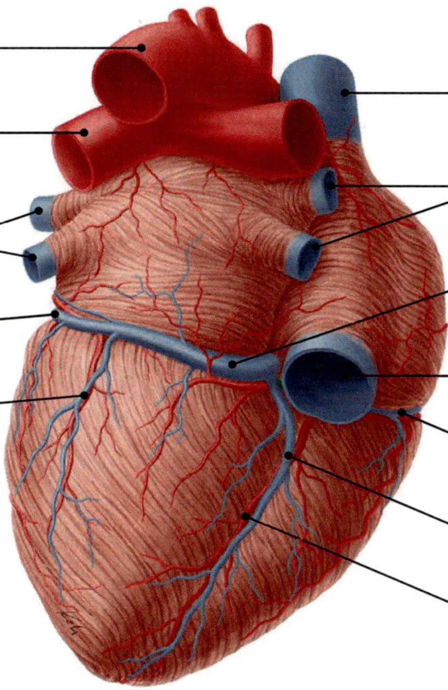

Fig 4.16 The major veins and arteries located on the posterior aspect of the heart.

The coronary arteries supply blood to the myocardium.

The two main coronary arteries you should know about are the left main coronary artery (LMCA) and the right coronary artery (RCA). You should also be able to recognize the coronary sinus, a collection of veins which direct the blood back to the right atrium.

The left main coronary artery supplies oxygenated blood to the left ventricle and atrium.[34] It also gives rise to the circumflex artery, which supplies the left atrium and posterior-lateral portion of the left ventricle, and the left anterior descending artery, which supplies the anterior part of the left ventricle and the anterior part of the interventricular septum.[35]

The right coronary artery supplies blood to the right atrium, right ventricle, sinoatrial node and the atrioventricular node. It also gives rise to the right marginal artery, which supplies the right ventricle, and the posterior descending artery, which supplies the posterior third of the intraventricular septum.

The coronary artery system can be subject to different types of pathologies which can give rise to coronary ischemia, angina, and infarction. An important aspect to know regarding cardiac valves is that they contain veins, thus preventing the backflow of blood in the heart.

Extra Medical Knowledge

The coronary venous system is main system responsible for the drainage of the myocardium. It consists of two major contributors. An interesting fact is that the myocardium contains around twice the number of cardiac veins than coronary arteries.[15] The following fact makes us understand the crucial role that coronary veins plays in the cardiac circulation. Indeed, coronary veins are responsible for maintaining the venous of the heart and they do so by thanks to their low resistance properties.[32]

There are two main contributors to the coronary venous circulation: the great cardiac vein group and the small cardiac vein group.[22]

The great cardiac vein originates from the apex of the heart and then ascends through the anterior longitudinal sulcus to reach the base of the ventricles. From the base of the ventricles it goes posteriorly merging with the oblique vein, forming the coronary sinus.[22] The latter then drains into the right atrium. The great cardiac vein receives blood from the anterior cardiac vein, atrial veins and veins of the ventricular septum.

The small cardiac vein is also called he right cardiac vein and is responsible for the drainage of the lateral and inferior walls of the right ventricle. The small cardiac vein can drain into the right atrium, the coronary sinus or the middle cardiac vein. It follows the pathway of the right coronary artery.

The Coronary Sinus is the largest vein of the heart in terms of diameter, lying in the atrioventricular groove. This vein drains directly into the right ventricle through the Coronary Sinus Orifice. The main tributaries of the Coronary Sinus vein are the great, middle, small and oblique cardiac veins.[22]

The Anatomy and Examination of the Abdomen

By Vasiliki Kalogianni

Introduction to the chapter

Welcome to the Abdomen Chapter!
This will act as your guide to understanding the basic anatomy of the abdomen and how it is related to the examinations you will need to perform for your OSPE.

The abdominal exam is not one you should be scared of. It is pretty straightforward in terms of skills required to pass the station, as long as you make sure to practice it many times. This chapter will include parts explaining anatomy and parts describing practical skills. The idea is to give you a basis that will make the examination more understandable and easier to remember, rather than make you memorise random movements you will have to perform.

Knowing how to properly conduct a clinical examination of the abdomen and getting familiar with a healthy patient is the first major step to picking up abnormalities later in your career. This is massively important as the abdomen is a cavity with major organs like the liver and gallbladder, kidneys and bowel, and major vessels like the abdominal aorta, and hence any problem associated with it may be detrimental for a patient. It will be crucial that as a junior doctor you are able to recognise signs related to abdominal diseases.

Clinical Communication

"I have been asked to perform an abdominal examination on you today. That would involve me having a feel of parts of your tummy and also listening with my stethoscope around those parts as well. I would need you to have your chest exposed for that by lifting up your shirt and, if necessary, bringing your waistband down. The examiner will act as your chaperone. Is that okay with you?"

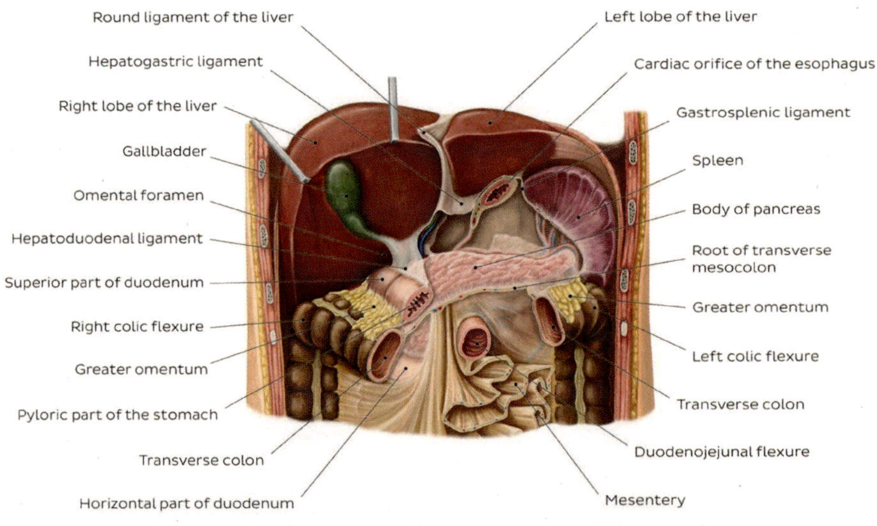

Fig 5.1 The contents of the abdomen in situ.

1 Division of the abdomen into four quadrants

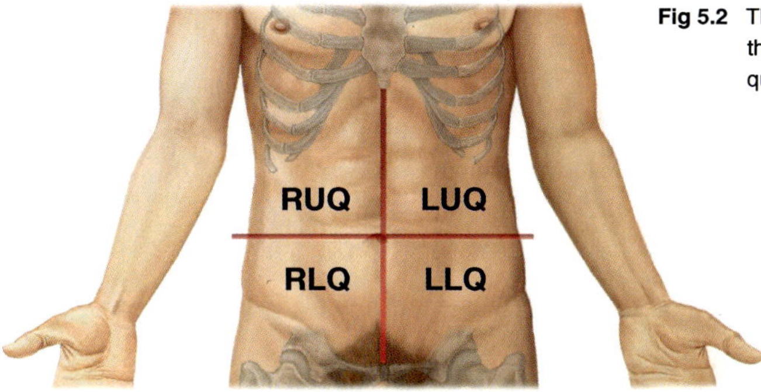

Fig 5.2 The division of the abdomen into quadrants.

In order to divide the abdomen into four regions, you must identify the vertical midline, which is a line passing between the xiphisternum and the pubic symphysis, and the horizontal midline passing through the umbilicus.[15]

These are the margins of the division, and the subsequent quadrants created are the upper right, lower right, upper left, and lower left quadrants.

Good Medical Practice

The mental division into quadrants is the "simplest" way of compartmentalising the abdomen. It is important as it allows for a better visualisation of the structures involved in a clinical scenario, such as when a patient has pain in a specific quadrant.[36]

Right Upper Quadrant	*Left Upper Quadrant*
1) right lobe of liver 6) gallbladder 2) pancreatic head 7) right adrenal gland 3) right kidney 8) duodenum 4) upper part of ascending colon 5) first part of transverse colon	1) left lobe of liver 2) left kidney 3) stomach 4) pancreatic body & tail 5) left adrenal gland 6) spleen 7) final part of transverse colon 8) upper part of descending colon
Right Lower Quadrant	*Left Upper Quadrant*
1) appendix 6) lower part of ascending colon 2) cecum 7) bladder (if very full) 3) right ovary and fallopian tube (female) 4) right vas deferens (male) 5) nerves and vessels of the right testis (male)	1) sigmoid colon 5) left vas deferens 2) lower part of the descending colon 3) left ovary and fallopian tube (female) 4) nerves and vessels of the left testis (male)

2 Division of the abdomen into nine regions

In order to divide the abdomen into nine regions, you must identify four planes:

Horizontally:

- The ***subcostal*** plane (L3) = line passing through the lowest margin of the ribs.
  - Palpate the costal margin on the level of rib 10 and once you get to its lowest point you will have found the level of the plane.
- The ***transtubercular*** plane (L5) = line passing through the iliac tubercles.
  - The iliac tubercles are superior prominences of the iliium that can be palpated posteriorly to the Anterior Superior Iliac Spines. Do not confuse the iliac tubercles with the pubic tubercles (which are found on the pubis of the pelvic bone).

Vertically:

- The two midclavicular (MCL) lines on either side.

The abdomen is then divided into 9 regions named as such:
Top row: Right Hypochondriac, Epigastric, Left Hypochondriac
Centre row: Right lumbar, Umbilical, Left Lumbar
Bottom row: Right Inguinal, Suprapubic (or Hypogastric), Left Inguinal

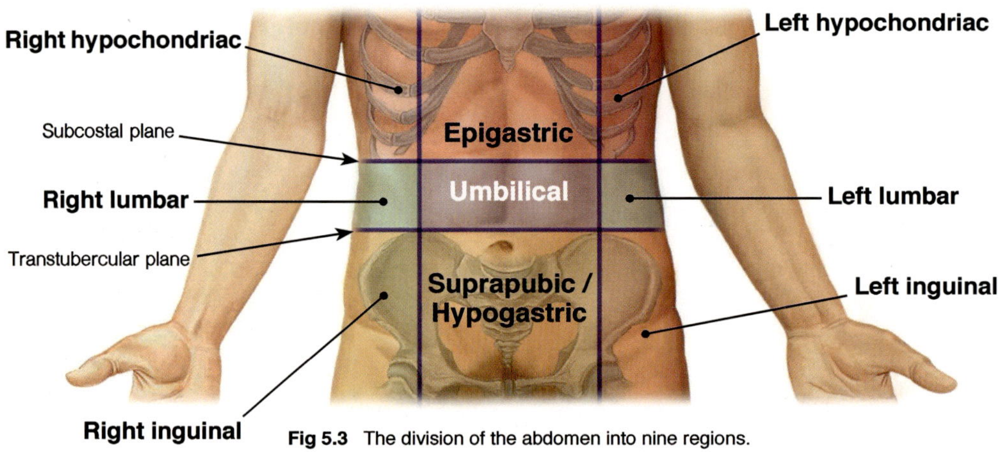

Fig 5.3 The division of the abdomen into nine regions.

Extra Medical Knowledge[36]

Right hypochondriac 1) small intestine 2) right kidney 3) gallbladder 5) liver 4) hepatic flexure of colon	*Epigastric* 1) adrenal glands 2) spleen 6) liver 3) pancreas 4) duodenum 5) stomach	*Left hypochondriac* 1) pancreas 2) left kidney 3) splenic flexure of colon 4) spleen
Right lumbar 1) ascending colon 2) liver 3) gallbladder	*Umbilical* 1) duodenum 2) ileum 3) jejunum 4) umbilicus	*Left hypochondriac* 1) descending colon 2) left kidney
Right inguinal 1) cecum 2) appendix	*Suprapubic* 1) female reproductive organs 2) sigmoid colon 3) urinary bladder	*Left hypochondriac* 1) descending 2) sigmoid colon

3 Structures of the digestive system present at the transpyloric plane

These structures are:

- Pylorus of stomach
- 1st part of duodenum
- First lumbar vertebra (L1)
- Origin of the Superior Mesenteric Artery
- Hilum of spleen
- Liver
- Fundus of gallbladder
- Neck of pancreas
- Hila of kidneys (in supine patients)

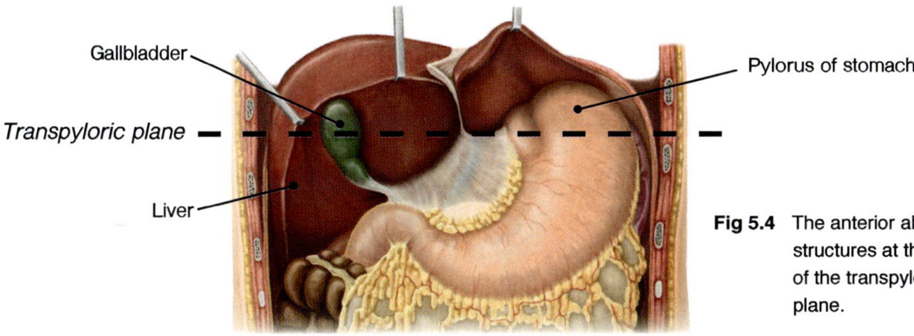

Fig 5.4 The anterior abdominal structures at the level of the transpyloric plane.

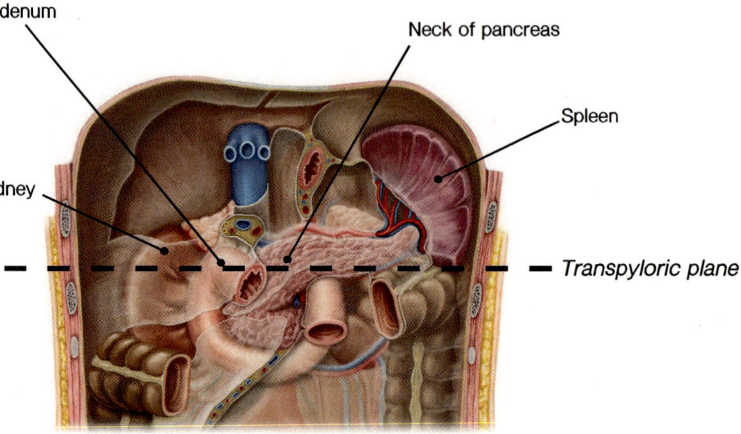

Fig 5.5 The posterior abdominal structures at the level of the transpyloric plane.

Good Medical Practice

You can come up with an acronym of your choice if that helps you remember the different structures.

For example, "Peter Pan Doesn't Like Golden Orange Hair" where:

P = Pylorus
P = Pancreas
D = Duodenum
L = Lumbar (L1)
G = Gallbladder
O = Origin (of SMA)
H = Hila (of Kidneys)
Etc.

Another example: "Grandparents Like Paediatric Doctors Preventing Kids Sickness" where:

G = Gallbladder
L = Liver
P = Pylorus
D = Duodenum
P = Pancreas
K = Kidneys
S = Spleen

It is important to know what structures can be found at the transpyloric plane (which is the plane at the level of the stomach's pylorus) as you will be asked to read MRIs, CT scans, or other diagnostic imaging. Although there is always some anatomical variation, these are the key structures that you should be able to find around the L1 level.

4 Liver, spleen, and gallbladder surface anatomy

The liver is mostly found within the ribcage in a healthy person, with the upper right corner being on the 5th rib on the MCL, the upper left corner on the 5th intercostal space (ICS) at the MCL and the lower right corner at the costal margin at the mid-axillary line.

Fig 5.6 The liver, gallbladder, and spleen in situ.

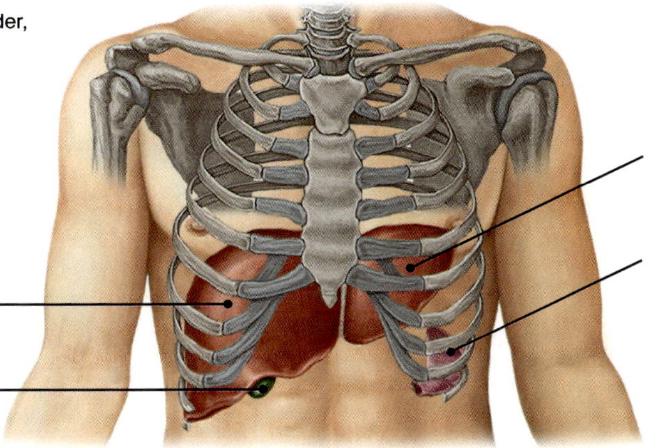

The gallbladder is found on the inferior border of the liver, where the rectus abdominis muscle meets the costal margin on the 9th costal cartilage (CC).

The spleen is found in the left hypochondriac region and spans across ribs IX, X, and XI. Its lateral margin is on the level of the midaxillary line, whereas the medial margin is on the lateral border of the Erector spinae muscles.[15]

In order to demonstrate the anatomical position of the liver and the gallbladder, you would need to find rib V on either side. In order to do that, show to the examiner that you are locating the sternal angle (indicative of the 2nd CC) and moving down ICS by ICS until you have found the fifth rib on the right and fifth ICS on the left side of the chest. The same advice goes for demonstrating the anatomical position of the spleen, when locating ribs IX, X, XI.
Please do not point at an approximate point and assume it is the 5th ICS or rib V without having visibly palpated and counted to check that you are referring to the right point.

Extra Medical Knowledge

In practice it will be important to know the normal borders of the liver as any enlargement will hint towards liver disease, cancer, or even heart problems that can, in some cases, be asymptomatic.[37]
Like the liver, enlargement of the spleen beyond its normal borders can be indicative of viral or bacterial infections, metabolic disorders, or blood disorders and they can sometimes be asymptomatic.[37]

5 Superficial and deep palpation of the abdomen

Before starting the palpation, you need to mentally divide the abdomen into the different regions discussed in the previous learning objectives, and you should always ask the patient if they are in any pain. If the patient has pain, begin palpation in the region furthest away from the region of pain. In practice, you are expected to also offer painkillers if the patient is in pain, but for the purposes of the OSPE's it is very unlikely that the patient will say that they are in pain.

Once you have done all the above, proceed with light palpation:

- Place your entire palm of one hand on the abdominal surface
- By flexing your metacarpophalangeal joints, press on the abdominal surface with, using mostly your fingertips to feel.

Light palpation allows you to identify any crepitus of the abdomen, which would indicate gas or fluid in the cavity, any irregularities, such as hernias or small lumps, and it allows you to specifically identify regions of tenderness. It always proceeds deep palpation, which is a more useful and informative form of palpation.

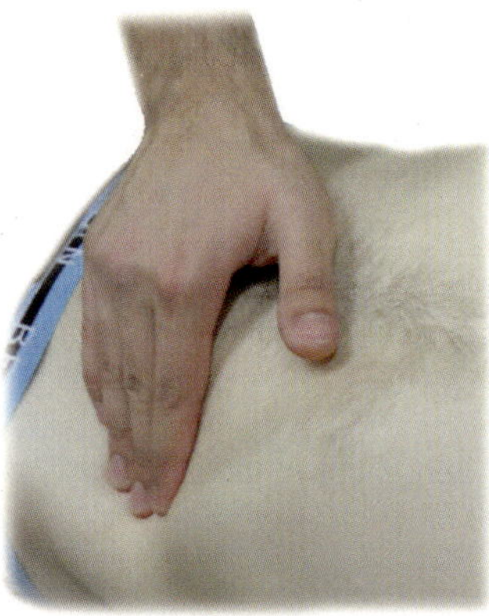

Fig 5.7 Light palpation technique.

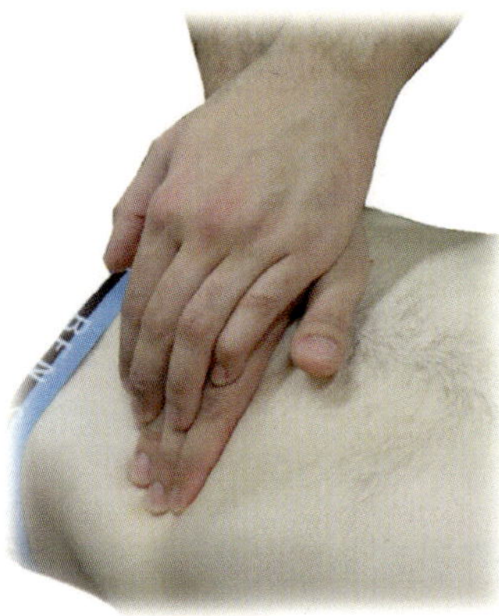

Fig 5.8 Deep palpation technique.

Once you have completed light palpation, proceed with deep palpation:

- Do the same movement as with light palpation but place one hand on top of the other for extra pressure and press deeper

Deep palpation is used for evaluation of a mass and internal organs, and also to further assess deeper masses and any deep tenderness.

Good Medical Practice

Maintain communication with your patient. This can be done in two ways. First, let the patient know what you are doing. For example, before moving on to deep palpation warn the patient by saying "I am just going to press a bit harder, please tell me if you feel any pain or discomfort at any point". Secondly, always look at your patient's face when performing palpation. Facial expressions will give away any discomfort or pain you might be causing the patient when they are too embarrassed to admit it. Practicing that on a healthy individual and making this a habit of yours will come handy in clinical practice.

It is important to maintain a structure when palpating, such as a circular or zigzag pathway. Please look at the example below, where palpation starts at the left hypochondriac region and ends at the right inguinal region.

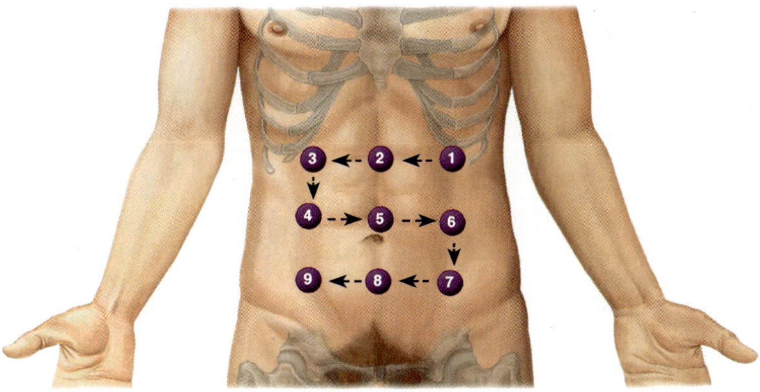

Fig 5.9 Suggested pathway for abdominal palpation.

6 Auscultation of the abdomen

In order to auscultate the abdomen, you need to use the diaphragm of your stethoscope and press it down onto the abdominal wall. Follow the same division and route as described previously for palpating, whilst listening for bowel sounds.

Since this is the OSPE, it is very unlikely that you will be faced with abnormal bowel sounds, which is generally considered to be the absence of any sound. Hence, if asked to describe what you hear, and you hear borborygmus (stomach rumbling), you are expected to say that you can hear "normal bowel sounds". State to your examiner that ideally you would listen for 3 minutes to conclude on the nature of the bowel sounds, but for the purposes of the examination – and how limited your time is- you should be doing it for 30 seconds.

Good Medical Practice

Just like with palpation, auscultation's purpose is to identify abnormalities in the contents of the abdominal cavity. When listening to the abdomen you are primarily looking for fluid sounds coming from the peristaltic movement of the bowel to ensure bowel activity. This is what is referred to as borborygmus, or stomach rumbling.

You are also interested in any blood flow or friction rub which would occur if organs were inflamed and swollen and hence rubbed onto each other.[36] It is generally harder to conclude that bowel sounds are absent and not just less frequent, hence why in practice you listen for 3 minutes.

Absent bowel sounds can be normal while sleeping, during specific times of the day or after abdominal surgery. However, they could also be indicative of peritonitis, which is inflammation of the peritoneum, and is accompanied by the inability to pass stool.[38]

It is important to know (and show that you know) how to use your stethoscope both in real life and in the exam.
You need to clearly show that you can work your way around a stethoscope and use it properly to auscultate the abdomen.

Make sure you place it in your ears the correct way (with the earplugs looking AWAY from your torso before you put them on – and so into your ear canals when you do wear them) and that you check by tapping on the diaphragm that you can hear sounds. If you can't hear the tapping clearly you need to rotate the chest-piece and try again. Make sure you do that to show the examiner that you are not pretending to listen to sounds – and to also familiarise yourself with your stethoscope.

Again, before placing the stethoscope on the abdomen, warn the patient! Say something along the lines of "I am just going to use my stethoscope to listen to your tummy. This might feel a bit cold, I apologise about that!" or something along these lines. Make sure you adapt these phrases to your own style of communication.

7 Palpation and percussion of the liver and spleen

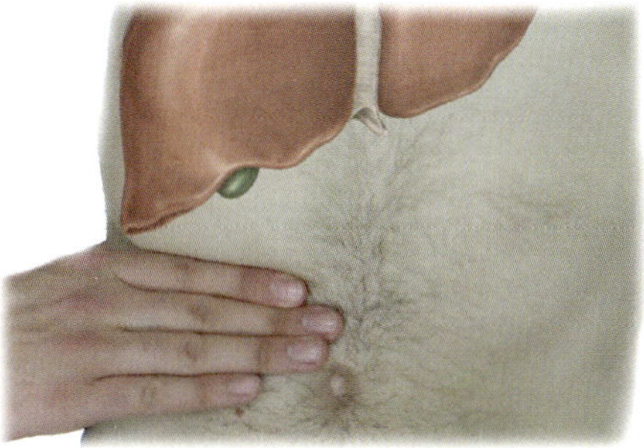

Fig 5.10 Palpation of the liver.

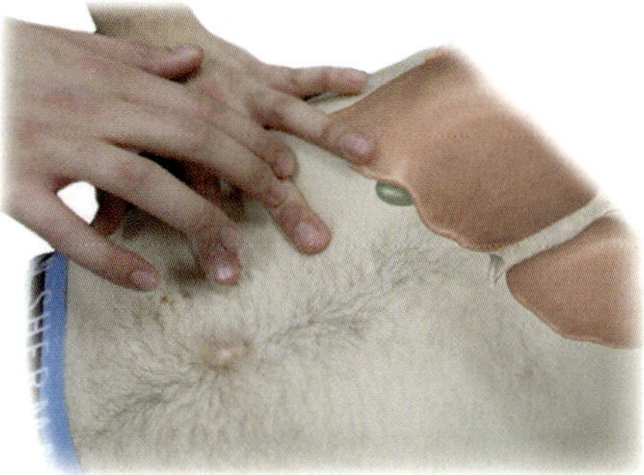

Fig 5.11 Percussion of the liver.

Liver

The clinical examination of the liver, as with almost all other organs, has four aspects; inspection, palpation, percussion and auscultation.

Palpation of the liver is done by placing the medial edge of the right hand on the abdominal surface. Start on the right inguinal region and ask the patient to take a breath in. As the patient is doing that, press firmly the abdomen. Work your way up until you reach the right costal margin, moving up each time by ~2cm. The reason you do that is because the liver is pushed down with each inhalation. If the inferior border was enlarged, you would feel it brush against your hand when the patient breathed in. You should not be able to feel the inferior border on a healthy individual. Hence, in the case of a palpable edge, you should be worried about potential hepatomegaly due to liver disease, like cirrhosis, or inflammation, like hepatitis.[37,394]

The process of percussing is based on the same mentality as palpation – that is to assess the liver margins. To assess the superior border, start at the second right intercostal space and work your way down until you hear the sound change from resonant to dull where you meet the liver, and from the right inguinal region up using the same method to assess the inferior border. Percuss by placing your left middle finger firmly on the area you are percussing and by tapping using your right index and middle fingers to elicit a sound.

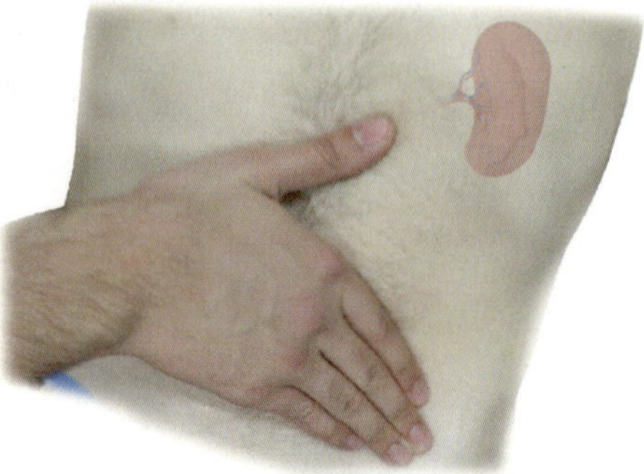

Fig 5.12 Palpation of the spleen.

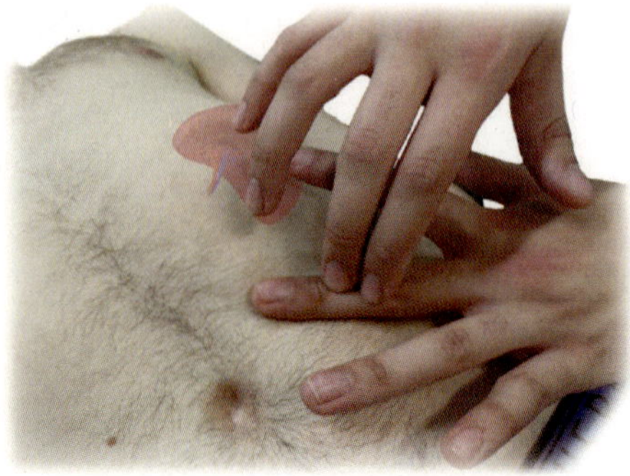

Fig 5.13 Percussion of the spleen.

Spleen

Palpation of the spleen is done in the same fashion as palpation of the liver, with the only difference being the route followed. The spleen enlarges anteriorly and towards the right side of the body, hence palpation starts from the right inguinal region and follows an oblique trajectory towards the left hypochondriac region. The same applies to percussion, which this time only assesses the inferior border, in the sense that the examination should start from the right inguinal region and advance towards the left hypochondriac. Lastly, auscultation of the left upper quadrant might reveal friction rub.

Good Medical Practice

Understandably, the liver of the patient is not visible so as to inspect it properly, so what is usually being done is that during the general abdominal inspection, the upper right quadrant is inspected for any obvious signs of enlarged inferior border of the liver, any signs of ascites (fluid collection) or any cardiovascular signs suggestive of cirrhosis or malignancy.[37]

An enlarged spleen should not be ignored as, depending on other symptoms, it can suggest liver disease, infection (such as in bacterial endocarditis), inflammation (such as in rheumatoid arthritis), or even splenic sequestration like sickle cell or haemolytic anaemia, all of which are extremely serious and should not be missed.[37]

8 Initial and referred pain from the gallbladder

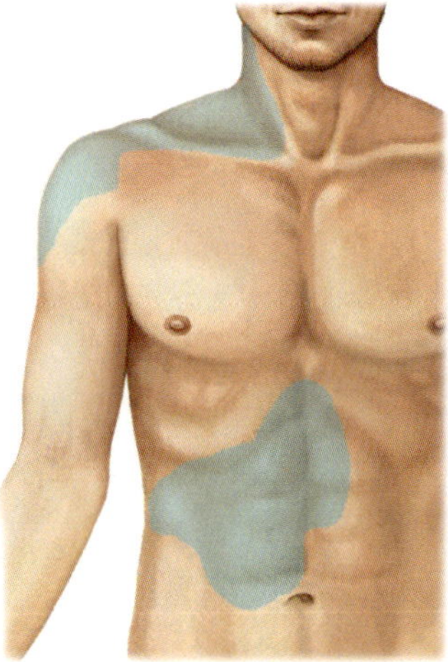

Fig 5.14 Anterior sites of initial and referred gallbladder pain, highlighted in light blue.

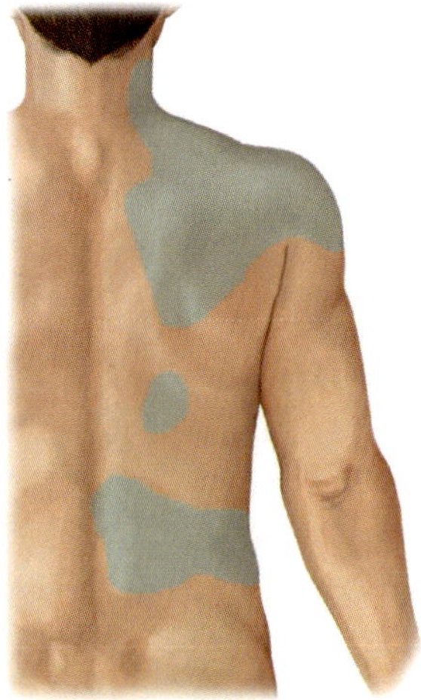

Fig 5.15 Posterior sites of initial and referred gallbladder pain, highlighted in light blue.

For the purposes of the exam, find the costal margin of the upper right quadrant (which would also coincide with the location of the gallbladder mentioned in the LO 4) and clearly show it to the examiner as the site of initial pain.

Referred pain from the gallbladder is found in the right shoulder.

Good Medical Practice

Recognising gallbladder pain in its initial stages is an important skill for any doctor, as upper right quadrant pain does not only indicate gallbladder disease. In practice, if a patient comes in complaining of upper right quadrant abdominal pain, then the liver and gallbladder are the first major organs to be examined through ultrasound and liver function tests.[40]

Furthermore, you might well be asked why gallbladder pain refers to the right shoulder as part of a follow-up question or just an "extra knowledge" question.
As the gallbladder is inflamed, it becomes enlarged and might push on the diaphragm, hence irritating it. This sends a signal through the right phrenic nerve, whose roots arise from the same place in the spinal cord as the supraclavicular nerve (C3, 4) - all bar C5 for the former- which innervates the shoulder. The supraclavicular nerve then gets stimulated and the brain confuses the location of the pain, thinking it is coming from the shoulder rather than the abdomen.[41]

9 Surface anatomy and palpation of the kidneys

Both kidneys span around 2.5 vertebrae (9-12cm long), with the right kidney being half a vertebra inferior in anatomical position than the left, due to the overlying liver.

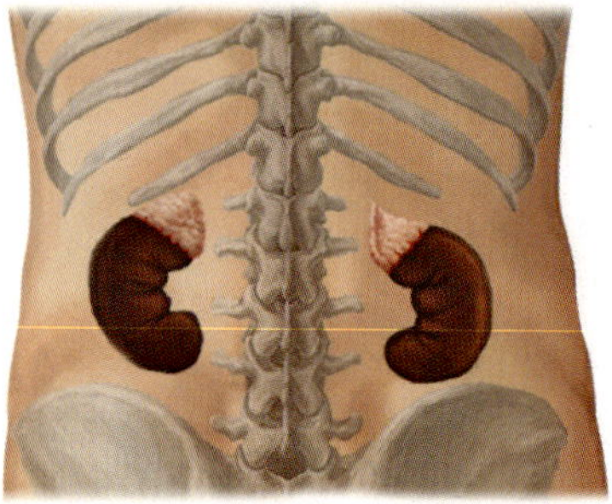

Fig 5.16 The kidneys in relation to the vertebral column and pelvis.

Key landmarks of the left kidney (which is half a vertebra superior for the right kidney):[15]

- Hilum of left kidney is at the transpyloric plane (L1), 4-5 cm lateral to posterior midline.
- Superior pole of left kidney is at rib XII (with the superior pole of the right kidney being half a vertebra below)
- Inferior pole of left kidney is 3-4cm above the supracristal plane (L4)
- Ureters descend (almost) vertically from hila to iliac fossae

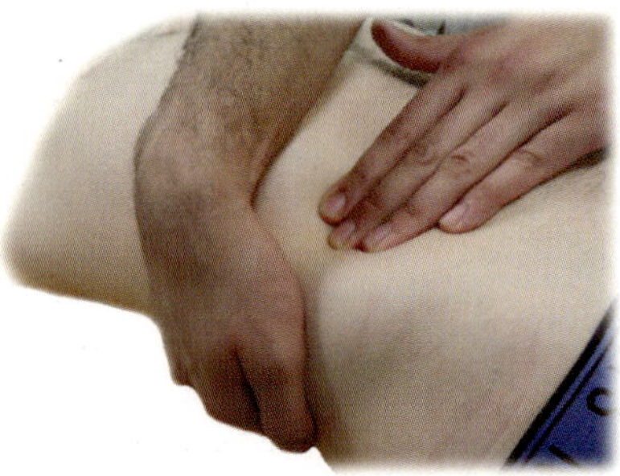

Fig 5.17 Balloting of the kidneys.

The technique used to palpate the kidneys is also known as "balloting".

To examine the kidneys, place one hand underneath the patient's flank with the palm facing upwards and the fingers in the renal angle. Use the other hand to palpate the anterior abdominal wall of the respective upper quadrant by pressing down just below the costal margin. At the same time ask the patient to take a deep breath in and use the left hand to bounce the kidney by flexing the metacarpophalangeal joints and doing a "come here" motion.

Good Medical Practice

Palpation of the kidneys is performed to check their morphology and position. In a normal patient the kidneys should not be palpable, with the exception of kids and very thin patients.

Palpable and tender kidneys show an abnormality, like stones, cancer, infection or blood clot.[42]

10 Lumbar puncture

In adults, the lumbar puncture is done between the vertebrae L3/4, in children between L4/5. To find the LP site, find the Supracristal plane (L4) and move up one intervertebral disc.

The patient can be either laying on their side with the knees as close to the chest as possible, or seating at the end of the bed leaning forward with the chin flexed towards the chest. Both of these positions help open up the inter-laminar spaces.

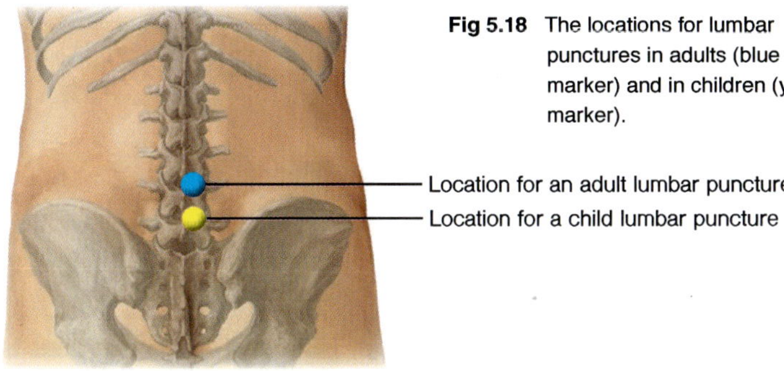

Fig 5.18 The locations for lumbar punctures in adults (blue marker) and in children (yellow marker).

Good Medical Practice

A lumbar puncture is most usually performed to extract cerebrospinal fluid (CSF), which is collected for the diagnosis of disorders of the central nervous system. It can also be performed to measure the CSF pressure – again as a diagnostic tool – and to inject anaesthetics or other medication.[30]

You would choose the L3/L4 space in adults to avoid injuring the spinal cord, as it terminates around the level of L1-L2 and becomes the cauda equina.[43] Therefore, this allows for a safer space for CSF extraction.
In children, the spinal cord actually terminates around the level of L2-L3, hence why you would need to puncture lower than where you would in adults.

11 Identify the bony landmarks of the pelvis

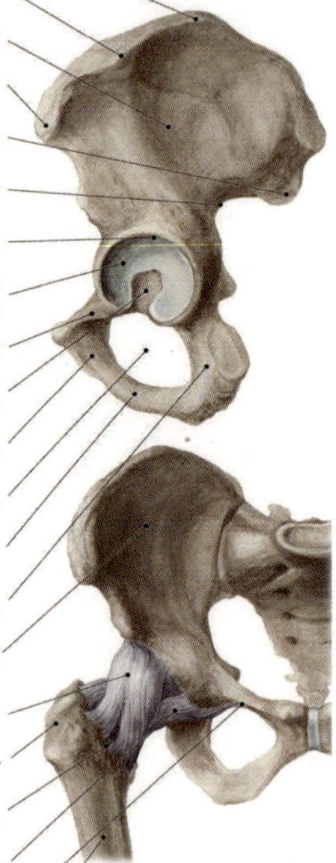

Fig 5.19 The bony landmarks of the pelvic bone.

You are required to know every labelled aspect of the diagram above for your pre-clinical curriculum. This is especially the case in the anatomy of the lower limb studies, and any aspect that has been labelled above is therefore fair game for the lower limbs station of the OSPE.

Therefore, although you might not be asked to demonstrate the iliopubic eminence in the abdomen station, it would be good practice to familiarise yourself with all the landmarks mentioned in preparation for the lower limb OSPE station, and your pre-clinical anatomy exams as a whole.

12 Features of the pelvic bone that differentiate sex

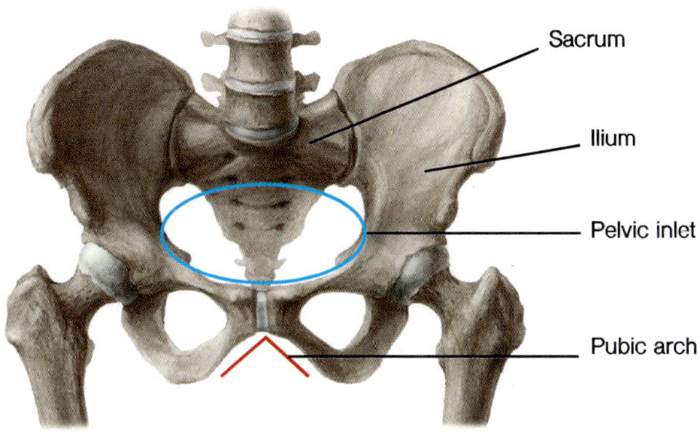

Fig 5.20 Sex differentiating features on the pelvic bone. Anterior view of female pelvic bone.

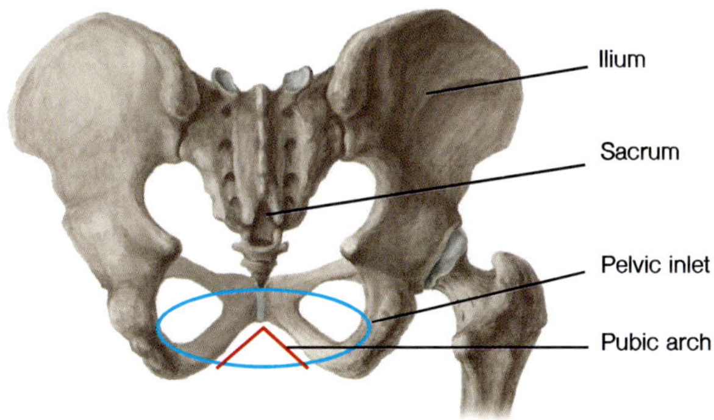

Fig 5.21 Sex differentiating features on the pelvic bone. Posterior view of female pelvic bone.

There are many features that you can use on a pelvic model to identify the sex of the pelvis. The following are what is required for OSPE, and they are the most basic of identifiable features.[36] A good way of remembering these things is to think about what purpose they serve. The female pelvis needs to be broader and wider to serve the purposes of childbirth, whereas historically males have a narrower pelvis that aids in locomotion.[36]

1) **Ilium** - Males have a more narrow and ilium compared to females, who have a broad ilium.
2) **Pelvic inlet shape** - Females have a wider and more oval-shaped pelvic inlet, as opposed to males who have a narrower and more heart-shaped pelvic inlet.
3) **Pubic arch** - This is the angle formed between the two inferior pubic rami, and in males, the angle is acute (approx. 70°).
   In females, the angle is obtuse (approx. 90°-100°).
4) **Sacrum** - Males have a longer and more narrow sacrum, as opposed to females who shorter and wider sacrum.

13 Identify the locations of the inguinal canals and rings

In practice, it is important to identify the location of the inguinal canal and rings because these are key locations for inguinal hernias. Hernias are protrusions of abdominal contents through a weak spot in the muscle layer of the abdominal wall. They are not life-threatening, but they can sometimes affect the blood supply to some organs if they happened to get trapped in it.

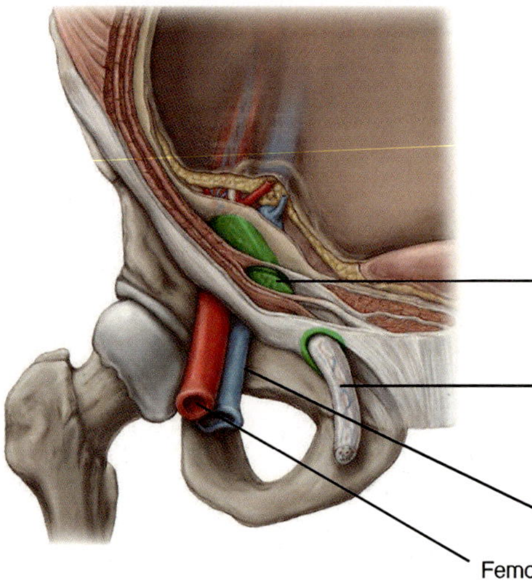

Fig 5.22 Surrounding anatomy of the inguinal canal, which has been highlighted in green for ease of viewing.

There are two types of inguinal hernias; direct and indirect. A direct hernia arises directly through the inguinal wall, whereas the indirect one arises through the inguinal ring and through the canal.

There are two inguinal rings – the deep and superficial – which constitute the beginning and end of the inguinal canal. respectively. The deep ring is located just superiorly to the inguinal ligament, midway between the ASIS and the pubic symphysis. The superficial one is located medially to that, in the medial third of the distance between the ASIS and the pubic symphysis, again superficial to the inguinal ligament. The canal contains the ilio-inguinal nerve and the genital branch of the genitofemoral nerve. In males, the spermatic cord also goes through there, as does the round ligament of the uterus in females.

14 The anatomy of the male pelvis

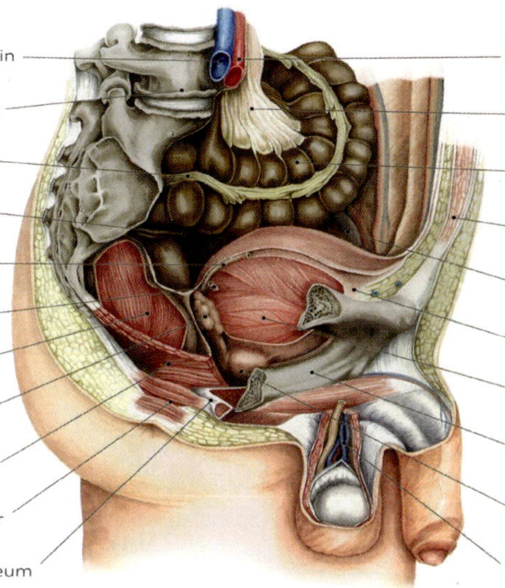

Fig 5.23 Anatomy of the male pelvis. Viewed in the sagittal plane.

As a follow-up question, the examiner is likely to ask you to:

1) Demonstrate the route of semen in ejaculation:

Sperm is created in the seminiferous tubules in the testes and is stored and matures in the epididymis, which is found on the former. From there, it enters the vas deferens and travels through the spermatic cord over the bladder and ureter, reaches the prostate posteriorly and joins the seminal vesicles. This collectively is called the "ejaculatory duct" and drains into the urethra which, finally, exits through the penis.

A good mnemonic to remember the route is SEVEnUP:
S: seminiferous tubules of Testes
E: epididymis
V: vas deferens
E: ejaculatory duct
n...
U: urethra
P: penis

2) Demonstrate the route of urine in micturition:

The route of the urine in males is pretty straightforward as it overlaps with the seminal route. Urine from the ureters collect in the bladder and travels through the urethra to the penis where it exits.

15 The anatomy of the female pelvis

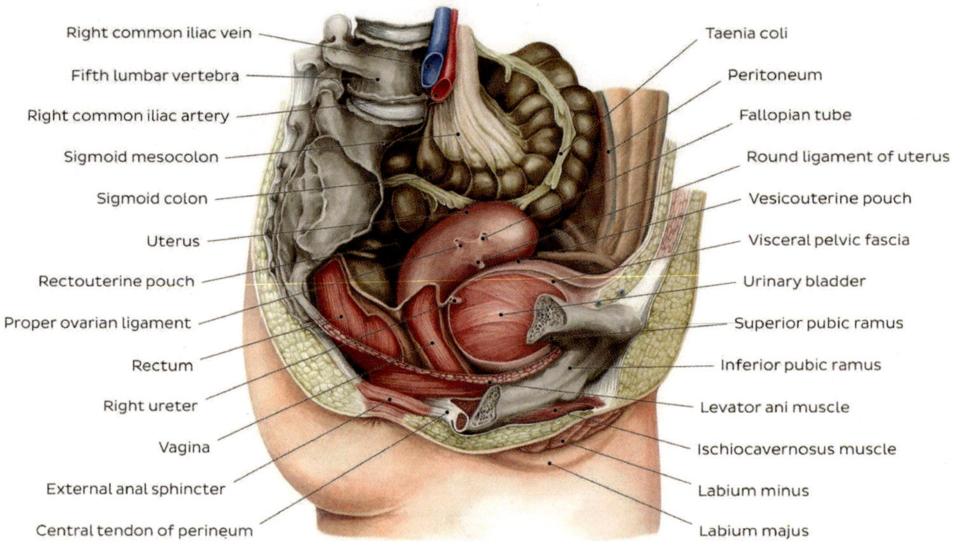

Fig 5.24 Anatomy of the female pelvis. Viewed in the sagittal plane.

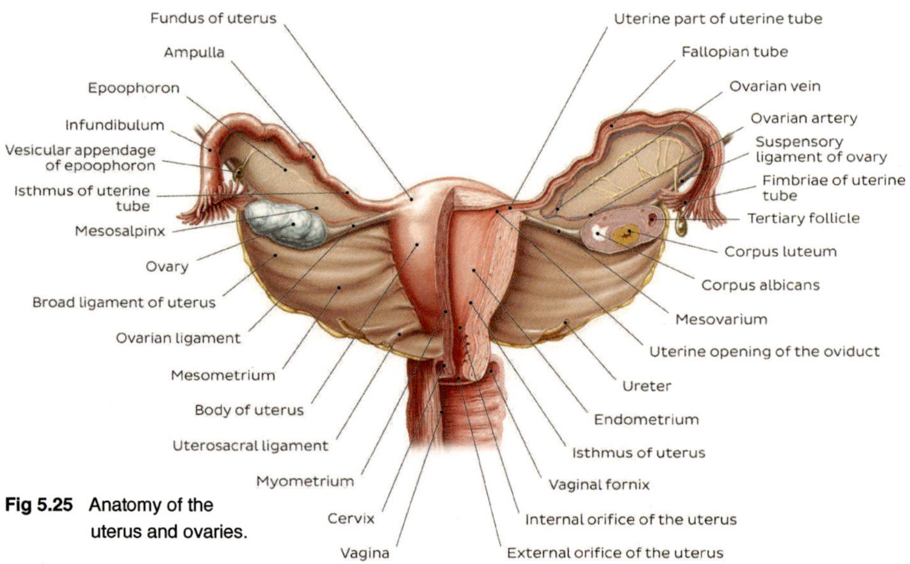

Fig 5.25 Anatomy of the uterus and ovaries.

Similar to the male pelvis LO, follow up questions could be asked for a female model:

1) Demonstrate the route of a fertilised oocyte:

The egg is created in the ovaries and is then released into the fallopian tube where it gets fertilised by the sperm (if present). It then travels to the uterus where it implants itself and remains there until birth.

2) Demonstrate the route of urine in micturition:

The route of urine is, again, pretty straightforward, but unlike in the male anatomy, it does not overlap with any reproductive procedures. Again, the ureters transport the urine into the bladder, and from there, urine exits the body through the urethra.

The male urethra is longer than the female urethra. This is part of the reason why females are more prone to acquiring urinary tract infections, as the length between external bacteria and the bladder is quite short and it makes it harder for the body to fight off infections. Another reason is that the opening of the urethra in females is closer to the anus than in males, and hence it is easier for pathogens from there to travel up to the bladder.

Head, Neck, and Spine

By Samuel Hammond

Introduction to the chapter

The Head, Neck, and Spine (HNS) portion of anatomy seems to be one of the more daunting stations in the exam; for one, it's a more clinically relevant aspect of anatomy since it includes neurological assessment and important spinal anatomy (and you will learn to understand how HNS pathologies, such as back pain, are hugely common).

However, the variation within HNS makes it incredibly interesting, and once you start to master the OSPE techniques, you'll start feeling more and more like a physician with each practice. Also, mastering a neuro exam makes you significantly slicker and more prepared for interactions on the wards.

As you'll know by now, the OSPE consists of 8 stations and HNS runs for 5 minutes like every other station, bar clinical communication. The stations can be in any order, but as with all stations, you'll be given the scenario before HNS.

This chapter will give you a breakdown of each HNS learning objective for the OSPE; provide you with what you need to know to score full marks in the assessment; and also some good medical practice (GMP) tips to allow you to form a solid foundation on which to begin your experiences of clinical neurology, along with ways to help you better remember facts in the long-run.

These tips are great to help clear up things and put your mind at ease, and occasionally they'll include something interesting medicine that you wouldn't have known from your pre-clinical studies.

Clinical Communication

"I have been asked to perform a head, neck, and spine examination on you today. That would involve asking you to do some movements and having a feel of your face and neck – would that be okay?"

1 The cranial bones and the pterion

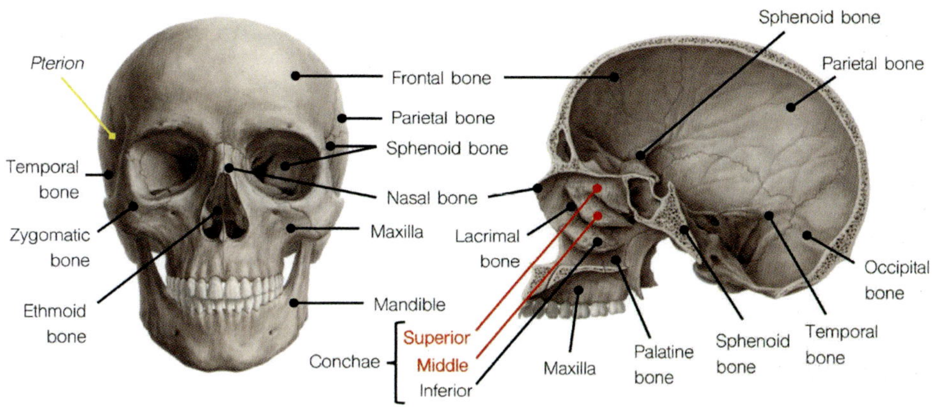

Fig 6.1 The bones of the cranium, along with the pterion, and superior and middle nasal conchae. The vomer has not been represented, but is described below.

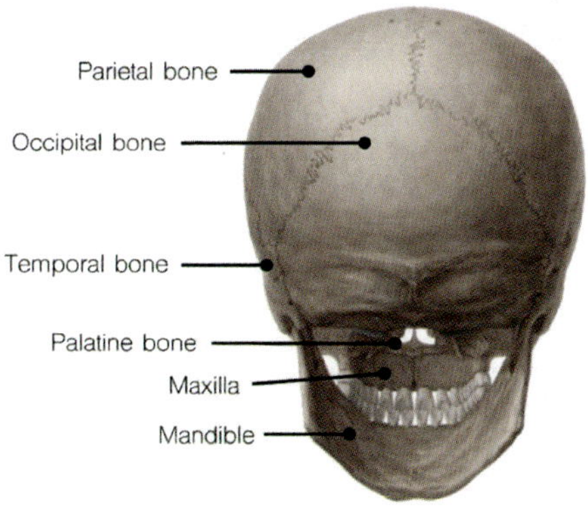

Learning notes

The absolute best way to learn bones and structures is to practice on an actual skull model. Make sure to effectively use your living anatomy time to practice this as much as possible.
Remember, the pterion is the joining of the frontal, sphenoid, parietal and temporal bones. The Pterion is a particularly weak part of the skull and since the middle meningeal artery lies below here, fracture or damage to the pterion can result in an epidural haemorrhage.[33]
Also, the superior and middle nasal conchae are not separate bones in their own right, unlike the inferior nasal conchae which are separate facial bones. They are just different parts on each side of the ethmoid bone.
Bones in the cranium: Frontal x1; Parietal x2; Occipital x1; Temporal x2; Sphenoid x1; Ethmoid x1; Nasal x2; Maxillary x2; Mandible x1; Inferior nasal concha x2; Lacrimal x2; Palatine x2; Vomer x1.
The vomer has not been represented in the above diagrams, but it has been labelled in **Fig. 6.4**. It is a bone in the mid-sagittal line that forms the inferior part of the nasal septum.

2 Key cranial foramina and their contents

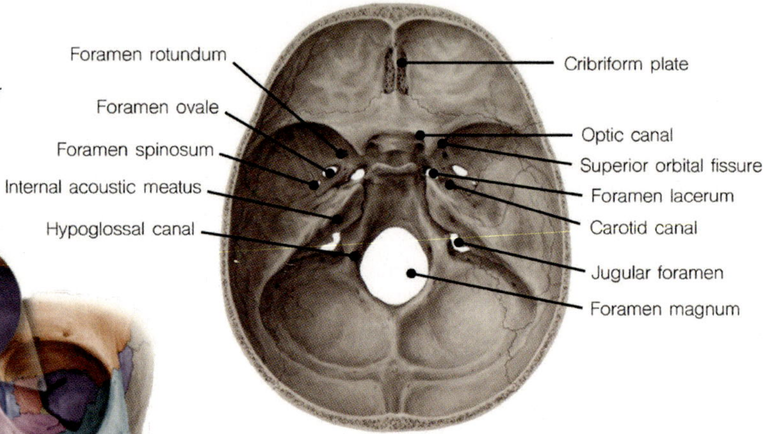

Fig 6.2 The key foramina of the cranium, (superior view of the skull base). The stylomastoid foramen has not been represented.
Diagram labelled by OMS.

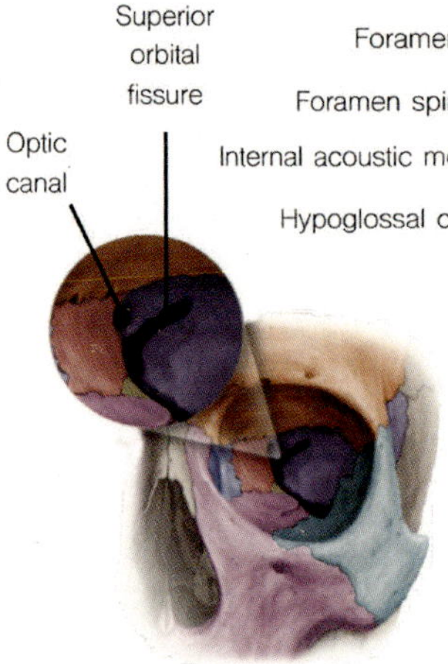

Fig 6.3 The location of the superior orbital fissure and the optic canal in the orbit.

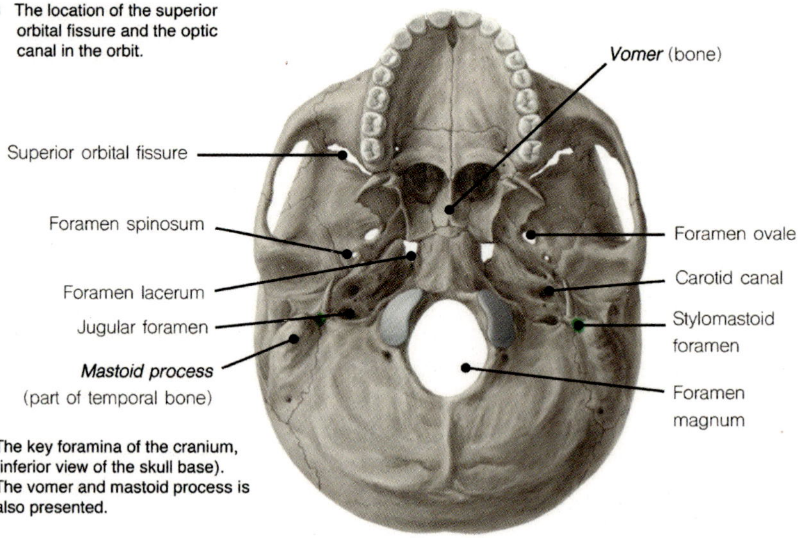

Fig 6.4 The key foramina of the cranium, (inferior view of the skull base). The vomer and mastoid process is also presented.

Foramen	Contents
Cribriform plate	Olfactory nerve fibres (CN I)
Optic canal	Optic nerve (CN II); Ophthalmic artery
Superior orbital fissure	Oculomotor nerve (CN III); Trochlear nerve (CN IV); Ophthalmic branch of Trigeminal nerve (CN V_1); Abducens nerve (CN VI); Superior Ophthalmic vein
Foramen rotundum	Maxillary branch of Trigeminal nerve (CN V_2)
Foramen ovale	Mandibular branch of Trigeminal nerve (CN V_3)
Foramen spinosum	Middle meningeal artery
Carotid canal	Internal carotid artery
Internal acoustic meatus	Facial nerve (CN VII) [*Entry into cranium*]; Vestibulocochlear nerve (CN VIII); Labyrinthine artery
Jugular foramen	Glossopharyngeal nerve (CN IX); Vagus nerve (CN X); Accessory nerve (CN XI); sigmoid sinus [*which becomes the internal jugular vein*]
Hypoglossal canal	Hypoglossal nerve (CN XII)
Foramen magnum	Spinal fibres of accessory nerve (CN XII); inferior portion of medulla; vertebral arteries; anterior & posterior spinal arteries
Stylomastoid foramen	Facial nerve (CN VII) [Exit from the cranium]

Table 6.1 The key foramina of the skull and their respective contents.

Learning notes

First of all, use the more obvious foramina to your advantage – the hypoglossal nerve is obviously going to pass through the hypoglossal canal.

Also, the foramina and the respective nerves which pass through them arise in ascending order; it starts from CN I at the 'highest' foramina when looking down at the base of the skull and as you descend down the foramina, the CNs are in numerical order.
Remember that the jugular foramen is the place where the sigmoid sinus for drainage of the cranium becomes the internal jugular vein.[33]

I would advise using diagrams to learn the foramina – knowing which nerve/artery/vein passes through the foramina is a start but you need to know the locations of each of the foramina too.

3 Sensory functions of the trigeminal nerve

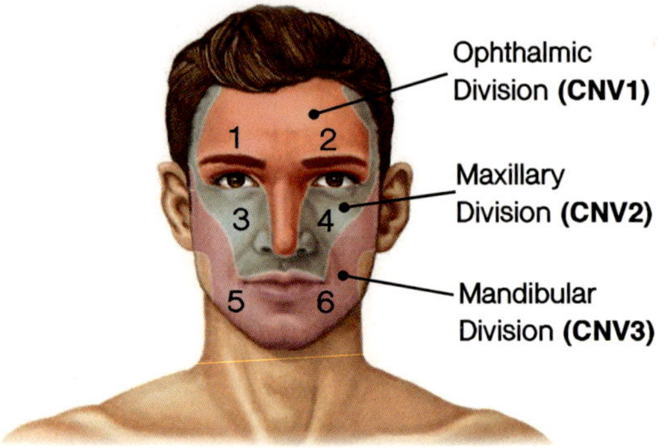

Fig 6.5 The dermatomes of the face, innervated by the different division of the trigeminal nerve, and the locations of where to touch the neurotip to test the sensory functions of CNV, in order.

Firstly, tell the patient what you're doing before you even pick up the neurotip;

"I'm just going to test the sensation of different regions of your face with a blunt pin."

You'll be testing the 3 major dermatomes of the face, consisting of the three divisions of the trigeminal nerve (CN V).
These are the ophthalmic (V1), maxillary (V2), and mandibular (V3) divisions of CN V, as labelled in the diagram.

The process of examination:

1. Ask the patient to close their eyes and to say "yes" each time they feel the neurotip touch their skin.
2. Use a neurotip to gently touch the areas as instructed in **Fig. 6.5**.
   Touch both right and left sides of each dermatome when examining before moving onto the next trigeminal division. As you will remember, there are two trigeminal nerves, like with all cranial nerves, present in a patient.
3. After completing the examination on each division of CN V, ask the patient whether the sensation they felt was equal on both sides: "Did that feel the same on both sides?"

Good Medical Practice

It's important to let the patient know what sensation they should be expecting before conducting the examination on the area of interest. Therefore, apply the neurotip on their arm or upper chest.

Equally, patient's must have their eyes closed when you test the dermatomes, so you are certain that they are feeling the sensation rather than seeing it happen. This might be very obvious, but you'll be surprised by how many people forget to this in their OSPEs and OSCEs alike.

Also, it's very good practice to check if there is any pain or discomfort when testing. This is for all examinations, and although you may have asked the patient if they are in pain during the introduction, it's good practice to ask them again before the first examination or any examination for that matter.

4 Motor functions of the trigeminal nerve

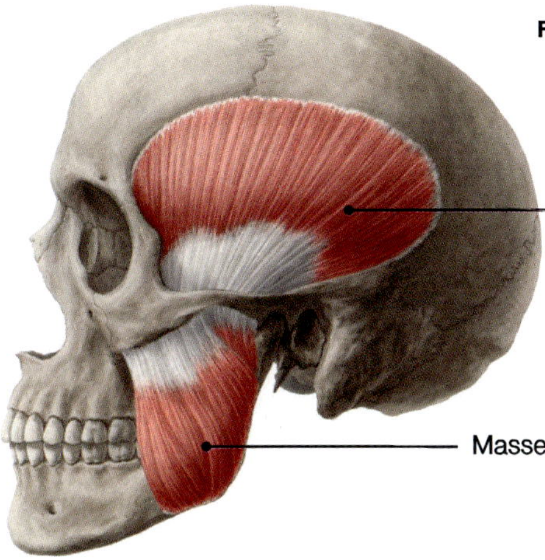

Fig 6.6 The muscles of mastication.

The masseter and temporalis are both muscles of mastication, hence they will be in a contracted state when the jaw is under tension e.g. when clenching the jaw.

Tell the patient you'll be feeling their muscle of chewing (and again ask if they feel any pain/discomfort).

Palpate the masseter anterior to the temporomandibular joint and palpate the temporalis muscle over the temples (pterion).

Good Medical Practice

Always feel on both sides of the face to check the function both muscles; any asymmetry in the muscles can be a sign of pathology.[44]

As mentioned, it's good practice to get into the habit of checking to see if the patient has any pain/discomfort during any examination – encourage them to tell you of any pain each time you perform a different test.

Medical fact: 'Trismus', otherwise known as 'lockjaw', is the inability to open the jaw or have a reduced range of motion and can be caused by the spasm of these muscles of mastication.[45]

5 Motor functions of the facial nerve

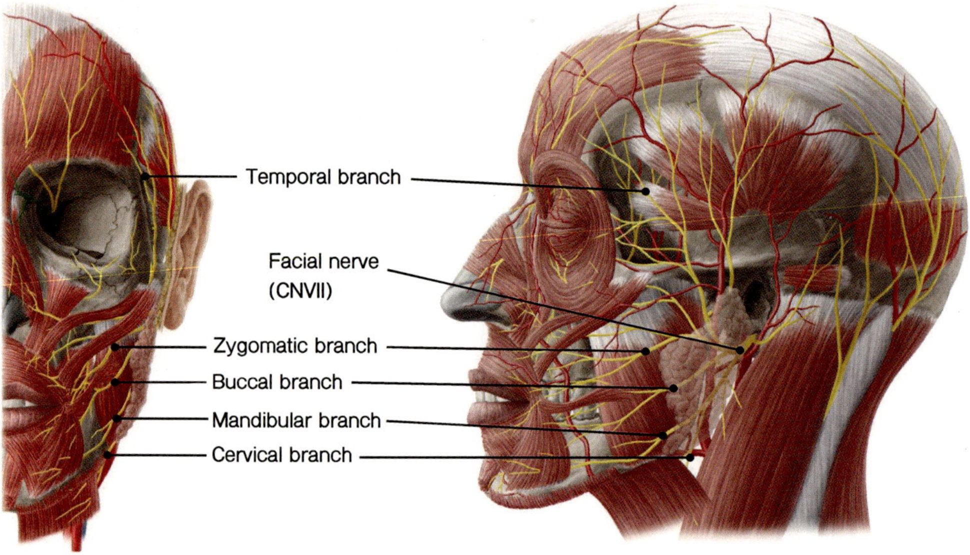

Fig 6.7 The branches of the facial nerve.

Acronym	CNVII Branches
Two	Temporal
Zebras	Zygomatic
Bit	Buccal
My	Mandibular
Coccyx	Cervical

The branches, and their myotomes, are tested by asking the patient to perform a series of facial expressions, as you provide some resistance to each movement. Don't forget to make the patient aware that you will be resisting their movements.

- Raise eyebrows/crease forehead – Temporal
- Closing eyes & squeezing them shut – Zygomatic [Orbicularis Oculi]
- Smile/reveal teeth – Buccal
- Puff out the cheeks – Mandibular [Orbicularis Oris]
- Grimace – Cervical [Platysma]

Good Medical Practice

You won't be expected have in-depth knowledge of which muscles control these facial expressions, but I've included a few anyway because it doesn't hurt to be keen.

The best way to explain this test to a patient is to tell them you're both going to pull some funny faces – it'll keep them engaged, make them comfortable, and they can easily copy the facial expression you're pulling.

Each time you test resistance to movement, ensure you tell the patient e.g. "don't let me push your cheeks in" whilst they're puffing them out.

I cannot repeat myself more about testing both sides! Remember, you're checking for anything unusual, especially asymmetry (although at the OSPE level patients are usually healthy and without pathology in the exam).

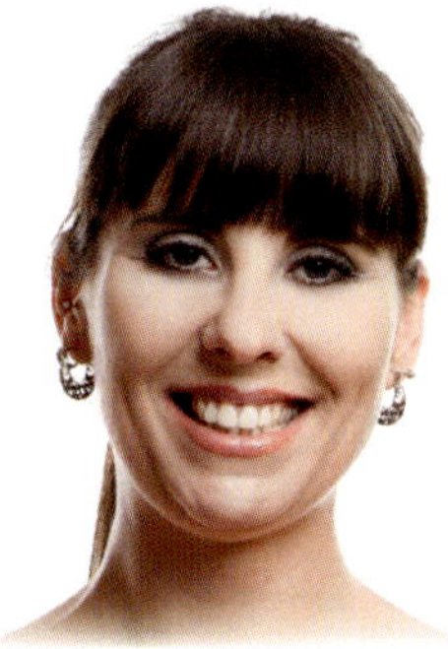

Fig 6.8 Testing the buccal branch.

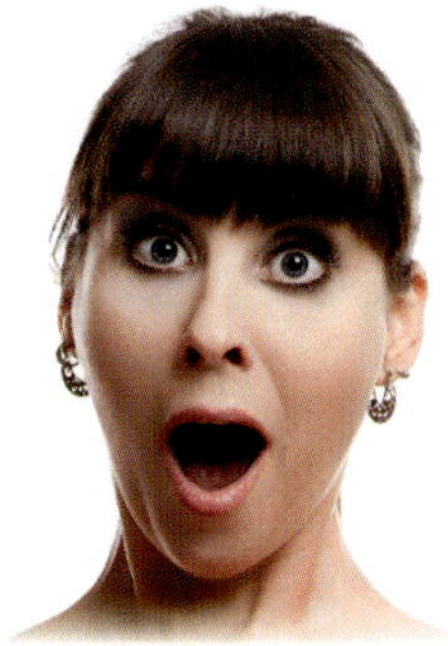

Fig 6.9 Testing the temporal branch.

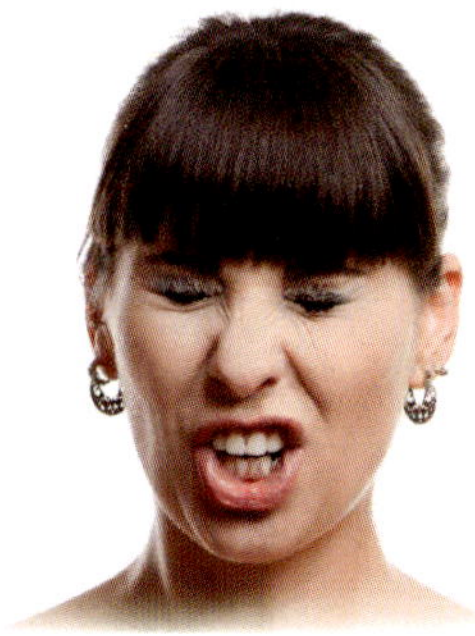

Fig 6.10 Testing the zygomatic branch.

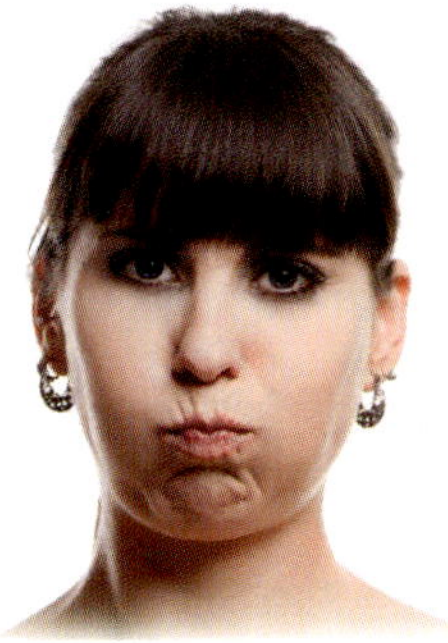

Fig 6.11 Testing the mandibular branch.

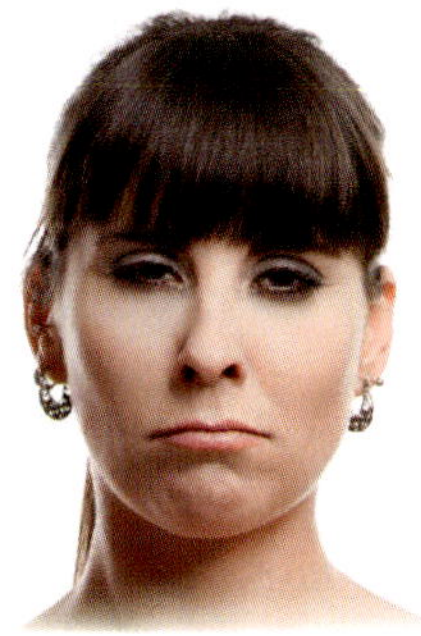

Fig 6.12 Testing the cervical branch.

6 Recall the testing of the glossopharyngeal nerve

Note that this learning objective asks you to 'recall', which does not require you to demonstrate anything. You just have to say that the actual test involves asking the patient to open their mouth, informing them that it'll be uncomfortable, and use a tongue depressor (basically a wooden lollypop stick) to gently touch the back of their throat to elicit the patients gag reflex. Please don't actually perform this on the patient in the OSPE.

Good Medical Practice

You should know the physiology behind the gag reflex even if you aren't expected to perform the test.

The sensory limb is mediated by the glossopharyngeal nerve (CN IX) since it provides sensation to the oropharynx and posterior 1/3 of the tongue.[46]
The motor limb is mediated by the vagus nerve (CN X).

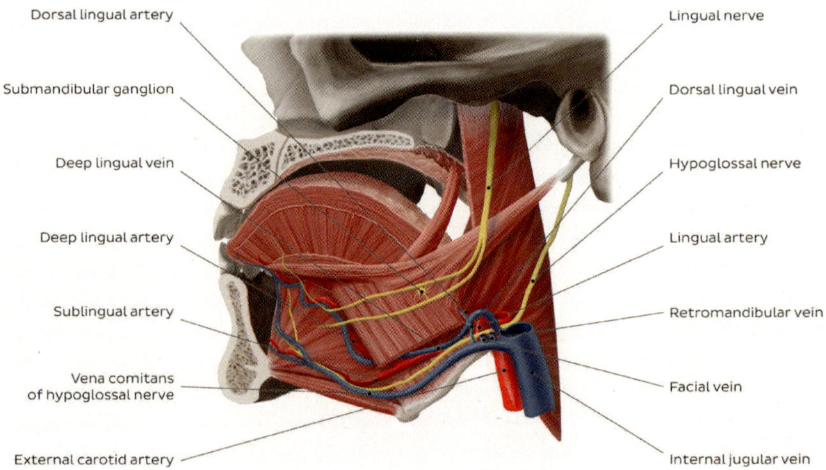

Fig 6.13 The innervation of the tongue.

7 Motor function of the vagus nerve

Simply ask the patient to open their mouth and say 'ahh'. This is done because the articulation of 'ahh' depresses the tongue and makes the uvula easier to see (a pen torch is recommended).

Then observe the elevation of the uvula, and check to see if there is any deviation from the midline.

Remember, uvular deviation is away from the side of the lesion.

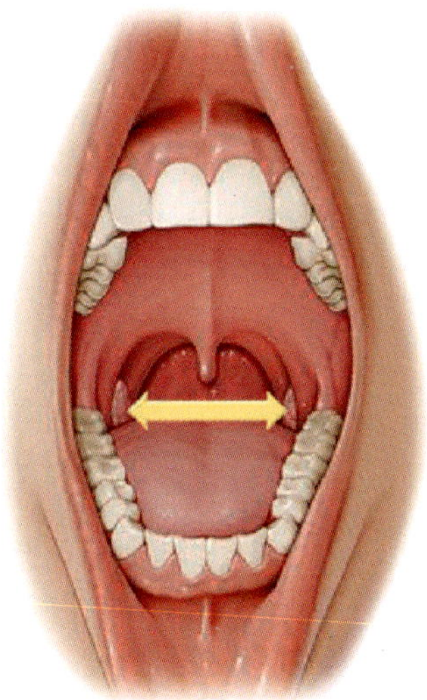

Fig 6.14 Observation of the uvula as an assessment of the motor function of the vagus nerve.

Good Medical Practice

As stated, this test is to look for uvular deviation since a lesion to the vagus nerve on one side will paralyse the muscles on the same side, resulting in the uvula being pulled by the contralateral muscle upwards and away from the lesioned side.
The phrase 'the uvula runs away from the wound' is good to remember.[47]

8 Motor function of the hypoglossal nerve

Simply, ask the patient to stick their tongue out (protraction of the tongue) and look for any deviation from the midline.

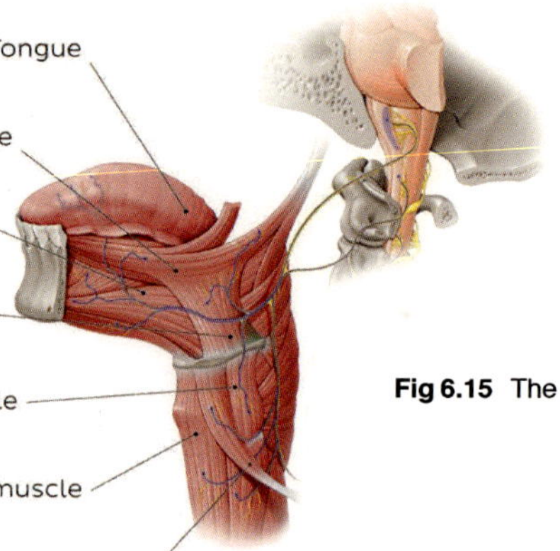

Fig 6.15 The innervation by the hypoglossal nerve.

Good Medical Practice

As the hypoglossal nerve is the only motor nerve of the tongue, this simple test is a good way of testing CN XII. The protraction of the tongue involves both the intrinsic tongue muscles and genioglossus, which are both innervated by CN XII. The Genioglossus attaches from the mandible to the bottom of the tongue. So, if you imagine that the muscle pulls the tongue out of the mouth, if one side is paralysed as a result of CN XII lesion, then the tongue will not be pulled on that side and as a result will deviate towards the lesion side (it lolls to one side). Remember 'the tongue licks the wound.'[45]

9 Motor function of the accessory nerve

This learning objective is very specific when testing the Accessory (CN XI) nerve.

To test the sternocleidomastoid (SCM), ask the patient to look to one side whilst you gently resist the movement of their head with the back of your hand. Repeat this process for the SCM on the other side by having the patient look the other way whilst you resist their head movement.

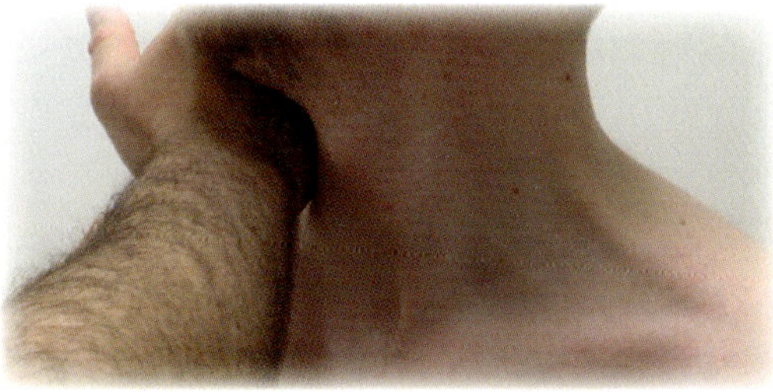

Fig 6.16 The testing of the sternocleidomastoid.

Good Medical Practice

To re-iterate, ask for and look for any discomfort the patient may experience when conducting this test.
Medical fact – the cranial part of the accessory nerve combines with the vagus nerve, and hence is considered to be part of the vagus nerve. It is the spinal fibres of the accessory nerve which innervate the trapezius and SCM muscle.

10 Extrinsic muscles of the eye

Innervation of the extraocular muscles

a. Superior Oblique - CN IV
b. Lateral Rectus – CN VI
c. Medial Rectus, Inferior Oblique, Superior Rectus and Inferior Rectus – CN III

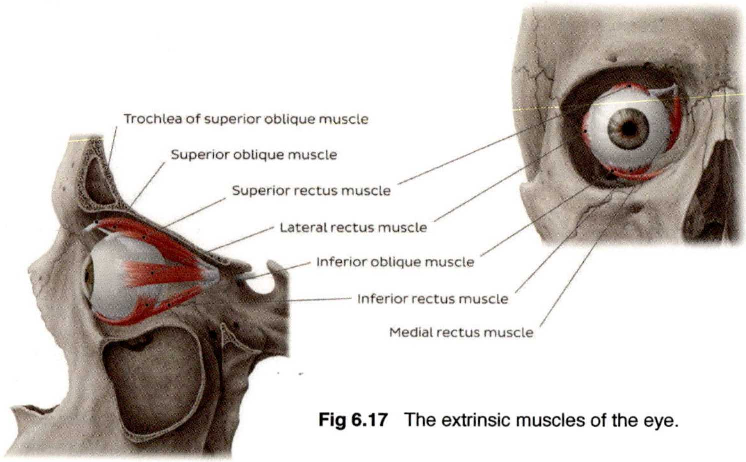

Fig 6.17 The extrinsic muscles of the eye.

Functions of each muscle [primary, secondary, tertiary action]

a. Superior oblique = Depression, abduction, medial rotation of eyeball
b. Inferior oblique = Elevation, abduction, lateral rotation of eyeball
c. Medial Rectus = Adduction
d. Lateral Rectus = Abduction
e. Superior rectus = Elevation, adduction, medial rotation of eyeball
f. Inferior rectus = Depression, adduction, lateral rotation of eyeball

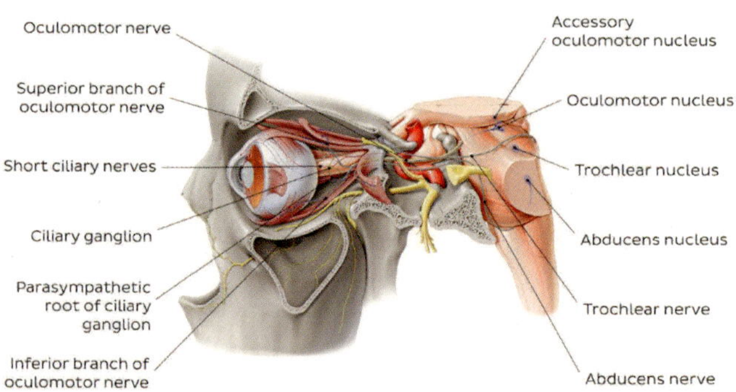

Fig 6.18 The innervation of the eye.

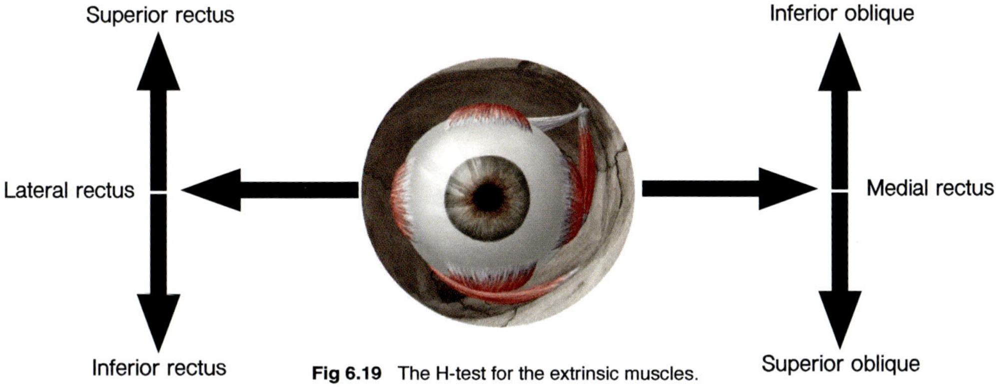

Fig 6.19 The H-test for the extrinsic muscles.

H-Test examination for the extrinsic eye muscles:[48]

1. Make sure to perform the test approximately 30-40cm in front of the patient's face.
2. Ask the patient to keep their head still, cover one eye, and follow your finger with the other.
3. Begin in the middle, move your finger fully to one side to abduct their eye (though perfectly acceptable to do adduction first) and move up, down, and then back to the middle. When you are moving up and down, place your finger in a horizontal plane because it makes it easier for patients with diplopia (double vision) to distinguish two fingers.
4. Repeat this by then moving your finger fully to the other side to adduct their eye, and then up, down and back to the middle.
5. The whole process should result in you drawing an imaginary 'H' in front of the patient (hence the 'H-Test').
6. Repeat this with the patient's other eye, whilst asking them to cover the eye that they just used.

Good Medical Practice

Knowing the anatomy of the extrinsic eye (extraocular) muscles, and their inserts and attachments to the eye will be invaluable when it comes to learning the H test.
Knowing their innervation is also essential. Repetition of the following phrase is a good way of remembering it: "SO – 4, LR – 6, all the rest – 3"
– if you're still struggling to remember, start with the lateral rectus; we know it's only function is

abduction of the eye, so it would clearly be innervated by the *abducens* cranial nerve. Equally, the superior oblique originates from the *trochlea* 'pulley system' of the roof of the orbit, and as such will be innervated by the *trochlear* nerve. Then all you have to do is remember that the rest of the extraocular muscles are innervated by the *oculomotor* nerve (for *motor* function of the eye).

Essentially, the H test is designed to 'trap' the muscle that isn't being tested since multiple muscles can achieve the same action. For instance, both inferior rectus and superior oblique can depress the eye. So, to test the superior oblique you should first adduct the eye to trap the inferior rectus – this serves to put the axis of the eye in a perpendicular direction to where the inferior rectus' muscle fibres insert (on the central, inferior surface of the eye) and as such traps the inferior rectus from its function.

With that in mind, when you perform the test make sure you move to the left/right of the eye enough to fully adduct/abduct the eye to trap the muscle (otherwise you don't isolate the muscle and multiple muscles will compensate with one another to perform the action).[48]

11 Test the ipsilateral and consensual pupillary light reflex

When light is shone into the eye, the pupil shrinks. This is one of the most obvious stimulus-response actions of the body.

1. Shine a light into one eye – check the ipsilateral shrinking (miosis).
2. Move the light away from the eye for 3 seconds.
3. Shine a light into the same eye – check the consensual shrinking off the pupil in the other eye.
4. Repeat with the other eye.

If there is both an ipsilateral and consensual reflex, the reflex pathway is intact.

Good Medical Practice

As with every test, explain to the patient what you're going to do in an easy to understand way e.g. *"I'm just going to check your pupil's response to light, so I'm going to use this pen torch to shine a light into the eye."*

Check for any pain and discomfort, as some people can be very light sensitive.

To avoid startling the patient and having them close their eyes, turn the light on and shine it on the side of their face, next to the eye, and then gently bring the light into their eye from the side. You don't just want to turn the light on whilst pointing it directly in their eye.

Similarly, don't shine the light in their eye for any longer than a few seconds; the reflex should be almost instant – any longer could risk damage to the eye.

12 Afferent and efferent arms of the accommodation reflex

The accommodation reflex involves the convergence of the eyes, constriction of the pupils (miosis), and bulging of the lens to very quickly change the focus of the eye to a near object. The test, which you aren't actually required to do, involves asking the patient to focus on a far object, such as a picture on a wall behind you, and then bringing your finger 5-10 cm in front of their eyes. You should give the patient a short countdown, so that they know to change their focus to the nearby object.

Afferent pathway for pupillary constriction:[49,50]

1. Ganglion cells in the eye
2. Optic nerve (CN II) [nasal and temporal fibres leave eye and nasal fibres cross at optic chiasm*]
3. Optic tracts
4. Pretectal nucleus
5. Edinger-Westphal (EW) nucleus [processing done here]

Efferent pathway for pupillary constriction:[49,50]

1. EW nuclei
2. Parasympathetic fibres along occulomotor nerve (CN III)
3. Ciliary ganglion
4. Parasympathetic fibres along ciliary nerves (CN V1)
5. Sphincter pupillae – constriction

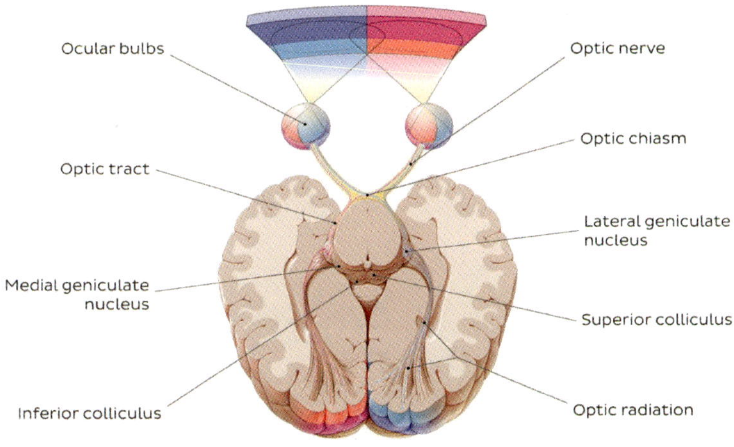

Fig 6.20 The optic nerve pathway.

Good Medical Practice

You must know the pathways here for both the afferent and efferent arms of pupillary constriction, even though the accommodation reflex actually involves two more actions as described above. It is also good to know that the convergence reflex involves the motor cortex since it involves extraocular muscles.

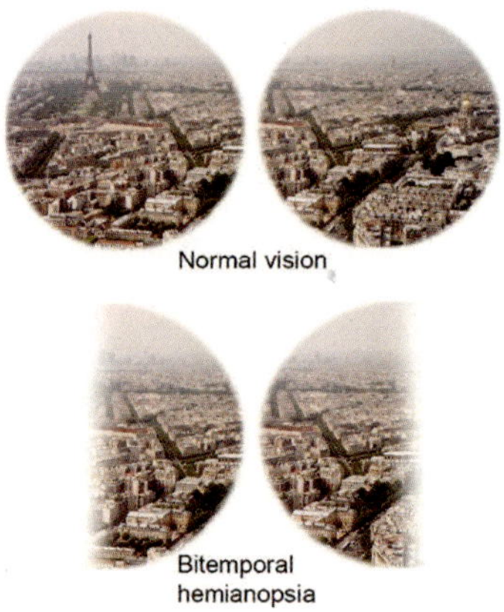

*This is essential when learning visual defect pathologies, as where lesions occur will help you determine which visual field will be lost. For example, compression at the optic tract leads to 'bitemporal hemianopia' where vision is lost in the outer half of both the right and left visual fields.[51] This is because the nasal fibres of the optic nerve provide temporal field vision and compression at the optic chiasm (where they cross) will cause vision loss.

Fig 6.21 Copmarison of normal vision and bitemporal hemianopia

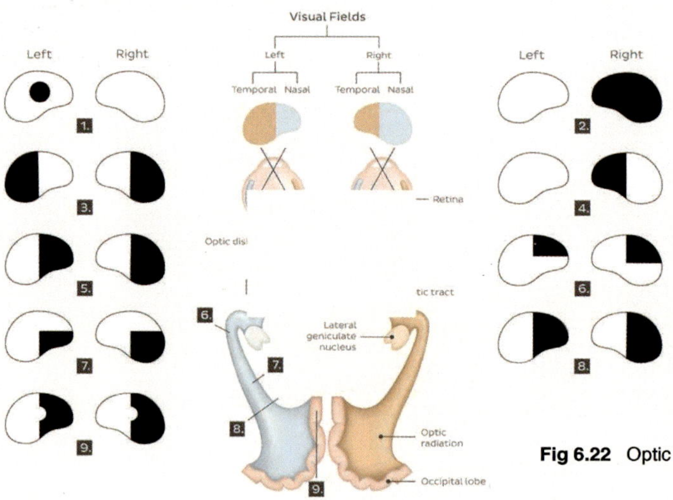

Fig 6.22 Optic nerve pathologies

13 Afferent and efferent arms of the corneal reflex

The corneal reflex is one you won't forget because the actual test involves placing some cotton wool on the sclera of the eyeball and produces rapid eye closure to protect the eye – fortunately you are required to recall, and don't have to do this test. Apparently, it's very uncomfortable for everyone involved.

The pathway is relatively simple and involves a sensory and motor component.

Afferent -> Touch sensation sent as impulse along ophthalmic branch of trigeminal Nerve, CN V1.

Efferent -> From Facial motor nucleus along Facial nerve, CN VII, to orbicularis oculi (quickly shutting the eye).[50]

Good Medical Practice

That's all the detail you need to know for this pathway, since the actual details are still quite unclear to us, but it is useful to know because it helps revise your facial dermatomes (knowing that CN V1 includes the eye) and also to know that one of the motor functions of the facial nerve is to shut the eyes.
If you keep forgetting, just link 'ophthalmic' division with eye (the ophthalmologist is an eye doctor).

14 Teeth examination

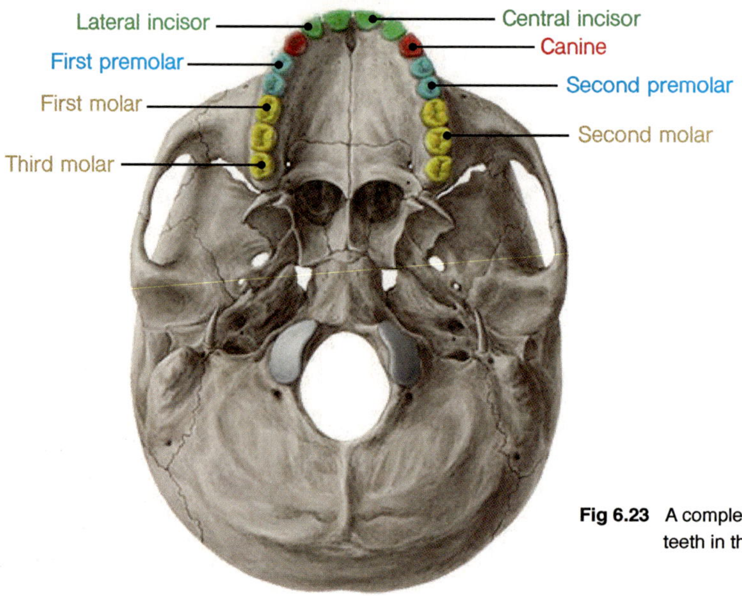

Fig 6.23 A complete set of maxilarry adult teeth in the base of the skull.

Ask the patient to open their mouth as wide as possible, and then whether they are in any discomfort.

Simply, count each type of tooth in each quadrant:
The easiest way to do this is to begin in a clockwise manner, starting from the top right of the mouth.

A complete set of adult teeth for each quadrant is as followed:

2x incisors
1x canine
2x premolars
3x molars
= 8 teeth in each quadrant (32 in a complete adult set).

Again, it's good medical practice to always look for, and ask the patient of any discomfort – they may grimace in pain etc.
Equally, don't use the term 'healthy' as a substitute for 'complete' when discussing a patients set of teeth; it can be healthy to have less than 32 teeth – such as in my case, I only have three mandibular incisors (weird I know, but still healthy!).

15 The hyoid bone, thyroid and cricoid cartilages, the cervical part of the trachea, and the lateral mass of the atlas and spinous process of C7

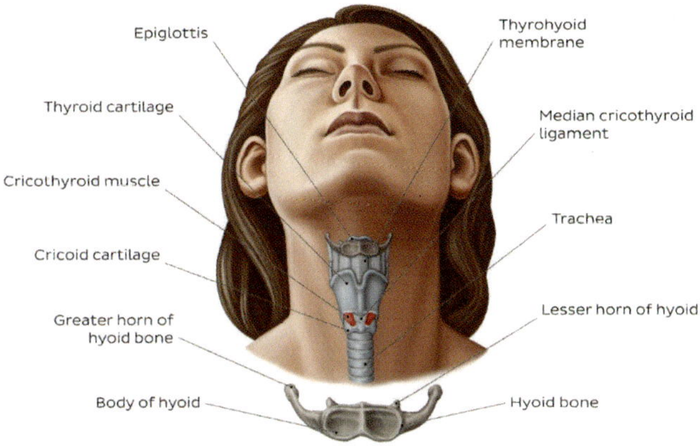

Fig 6.24 The larynx and the hyoid bone.

Fig 6.25 A cadaveric crycothyroid.

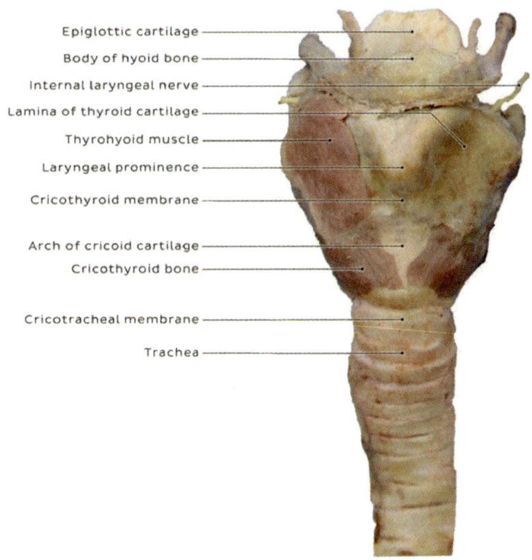

This will involve palpation of the neck.

As you know, C7 is the vertebrae prominens and is a good frame of reference for the other structures in this LO, since they're all found above C7. Place your index finger on the thyroid cartilage, and then ask the patient to swallow. You will feel the hyoid move up and down. Try this again, but with your index finger and thumb in a pincer position, 2cm superior to the thyroid cartilage.
This is how you will palpate the hyoid.

The laryngeal prominence is a helpful landmark because it's between the superior thyroid cartilage and the inferior cricoid cartilage. It is formed by the thyroid cartilage and is essentially the angle at which the thyroid cartilage surround the larynx. The thyroid isthmus is the aspect of the thyroid that separates it's 'wings'. The thyroid is found below the cricoid cartilage.

The lateral mass of the atlas can be found between the mastoid processes (inferior part of temporal bone) and the ramus of the mandible (the vertical aspect).

To summarise, the easiest way to approach palation of anterior midline neck structures is to start with the laryngeal prominence. Above this and lateral to this is the superior aspect of the thyroid cartilage. Even further above is the hyoid bone. The next palpable structure below the prominence is the cricoid cartilage. Beyond this is the thyroid, the isthmus is palpable in the midline and thyroid lobes are palpable more laterally.

16 Tracheostomy and cricothyroidotomy

In the event of airway blockage/collapse, often seen in trauma or extreme allergic reactions, these two similar but discernible interventions can gain life-saving ventilatory access to the lungs.

Cricothyroidotomy (also known as laryngotomy) – Transverse incision is made between the cricoid and thyroid cartilages, which are both palpable structures, into the cricothyroid membrane (also known as the median cricothyroid ligament).[52]

Tracheostomy – Transverse incision made between the cartilage rings of trachea (usually 2nd & 3rd rings); palpable below the cricoid cartilage. Note that the thyroid isthmus (tissue that bridges the lobes of thyroid) can be divided for better access.[52]

Good Medical Practice

Both procedures allow access to the airway which, as you know, is the first system to focus on in basic life support (DRABC). Therefore, these procedures can mean the difference between life and death for a patient. Cricothyroidotomy is more often used in emergency situations due to the ease of locating and piercing the membrane – however, as you'll remember, the whole larynx displaces during swallowing, and so the airway created during the procedure moves too – giving rise to a number of complications.

Hence, tracheostomy is often preferred for temporary intubation or for permanent, long-lasting airway access. It can also be done as an elective surgery under general anaesthetic; since the higher complexity of the procedure requires greater control.

17 External auditory meatus and eardrum

The external acoustic meatus begins at the opening of the ear canal and ends at the tympanic membrane (eardrum). The features of the tympanic membrane can be observed using an otoscope – an instrument that uses lenses and light to illuminate.

Fig 6.26 Outer ear and auditory tube.

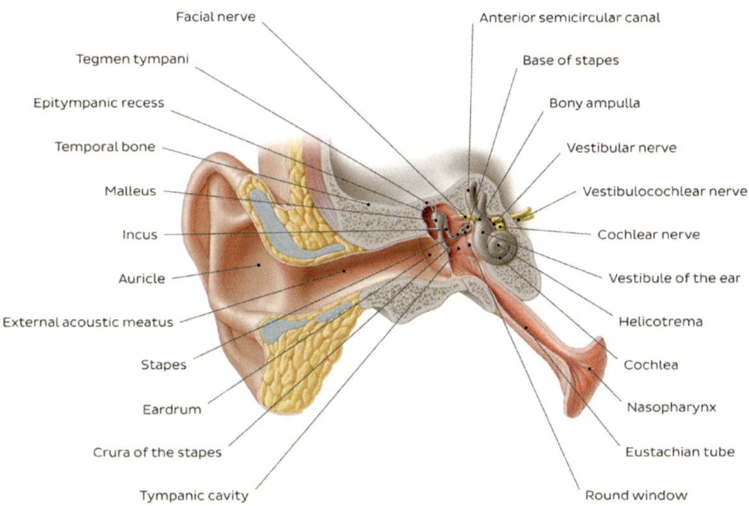

Good Medical Practice

You'll see the 'cone of light' at roughly 5 o' clock when viewing the membrane – it simply occurs due to light from the otoscope reflecting from the tympanic membrane.[53]

18 The carotid pulse

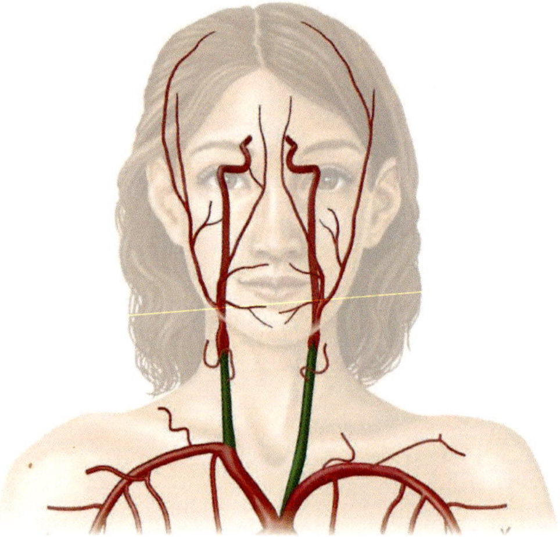

Fig 6.27 The common carotid artery.

The carotid pulse arises from the common carotid artery and can be found at the anterior border of the SCM at the level of the superior border of the laryngeal prominence (Adam's apple).

Good Medical Practice

To see the anterior border of the SCM, ask the patient to look to one side. Then place your finger at the anterior border of the SCM at the level of the laryngeal prominence and ask the patient to face forward again. Only take the pulse when the patient faces forward since the medial head of the SCM will cover the pulse when the patient is looking to the side. Pulses are best felt by pushing against a bony structure, and in this case, directly posterior onto the transverse process of the adjacent cervical vertebra.

Finally, please avoid taking the carotid pulse on both sides simultaneously. You'll know from blood supply lectures that the common carotids are extremely important in supplying blood to the head & brain, and the patient can faint if you occlude both arteries at the same time, which really won't look good in your OSPE.

19 Palpation of the cervical lymph nodes

Firstly, inform the patient you're going to "feel for some glands in the jaw and neck" or "check for any lumps in the neck". Ask them to inform you if they feel any pain or discomfort.

Always palpate the nodes from behind the patient (where possible).

The palpation technique is crucial here – move your fingers along in circular motions and don't lift them off of the patient – you can miss nodes very easily if you aren't in constant contact with the patient

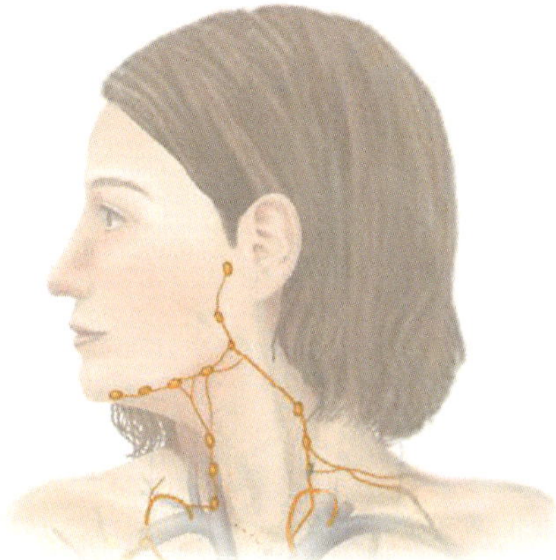

Fig 6.28 The cervical lymph nodes.

Good Medical Practice

There's no required order to palpating the nodes but you'll find it easier to start below the jaw (submental), and work your way posteriorly to the submandibular nodes, and then head down along the anterior border of the SCM feeling for the paratracheal nodes, and then the anterior cervical lymph nodes. Now feel the supraclavicular nodes and begin heading back up along the posterior border of the SCM towards the pre-auricular nodes. Palpate above the ears and back down to the post auricular nodes, move down to the posterior cervical nodes and finally medial to the occipital nodes.

This is the method I use, and you'll be told lots of different ones but find the technique that works for you – just remember to keep contact, use a circular motion to palpate and don't miss any of the node groups!

20 Central line insertion into the internal jugular vein

The internal jugular vein runs laterally to the common carotid. For central line access, a triangle in the neck is used. This triangle is defined by the medial, sternal head of the SCM; the medial third of the clavicle and the lateral, clavicular head of the SCM. The superior apex of the triangle is used as the insertion point for the needle.

- Needle inserted at 30˚ angle
- Needle directed towards ipsilateral nipple

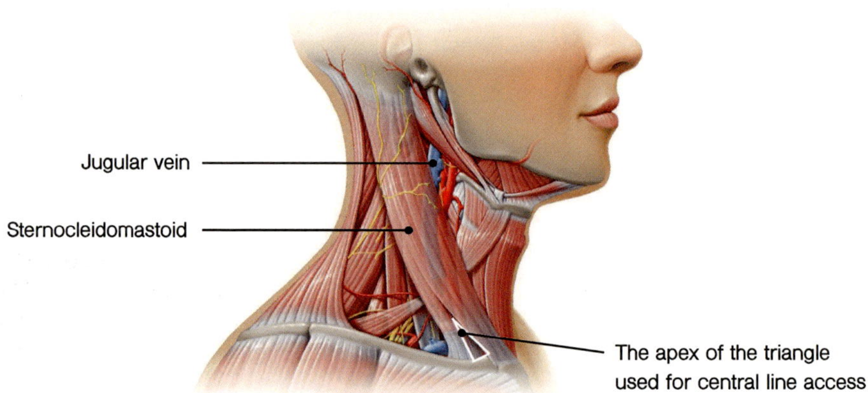

Fig 6.29 The location used for jugular vein central line access.

Good Medical Practice

In clinical practice, you may be asked to explain why right-sided jugular venous access is preferred. The right internal jugular vein is wider in diameter and often more superficial than the left internal jugular vein and so access is easier (and therefore safer).[54]

21 Anterior and posterior triangles of the neck and the jugular vein

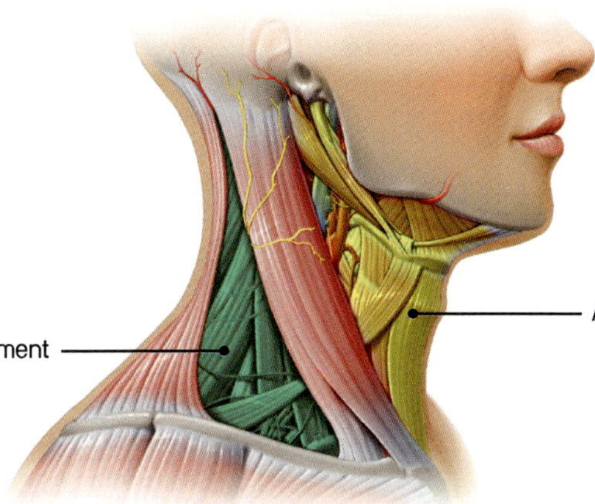

Fig 6.30 The triangles of the neck.

Anterior Triangle Boundaries:[33]

- [*medially*] Midline of neck
- [*superiorly*] Inferior border of mandible
- [*laterally*] Anterior border of SCM

Posterior Triangle Boundaries:[33]

- [*medially*] Posterior border of SCM
- [*laterally*] Anterior border of trapezius
- [*inferiorly*] Middle 1/3 of clavicle

Anterior Triangle Contents:[33]

1. Hyoid bone
2. Common carotid artery
3. Internal jugular vein
4. Supra-hyoid muscles x4 (stylohyoid, digastric, mylohyoid, geniohyoid)
5. Infrahyoid muscles x4 (omohyoid, sternohyoid, thyrohyoid, sternothyroid)

Posterior Triangle Contents:[33]

1. External jugular vein
2. Subclavian vein
3. Subclavian artery
4. Trunks of brachial plexus
5. Phrenic nerve
6. Vagus nerve
7. Spinal accessory nerve

The internal jugular vein runs parallel and lateral to common carotid artery.

The external jugular vein runs from the angle of mandible to the middle of the clavicle.

Good Medical Practice

The key to remembering the strap muscles is to understand where the name comes from e.g. 'geniohyoid' – 'genio' meaning chin and 'hyoid' meaning the hyoid bone.

22 Bones of the nasal cavity

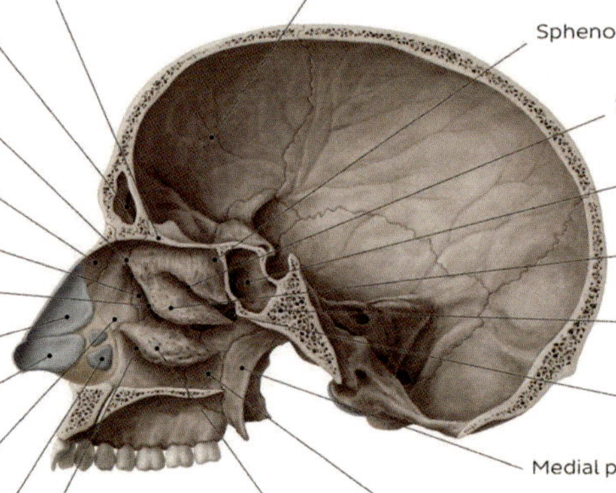

Fig 6.31 The bones of the lateral wall of the nasal cavity.

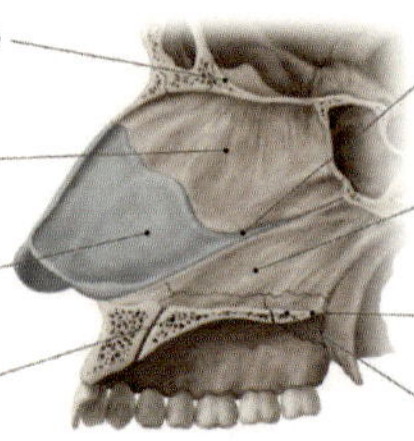

Fig 6.32 The bones of the medial wall of the nasal cavity.

Good Medical Practice

The nasal septum consists of the vomer bone inferiorly and the perpendicular plate of ethmoid bone superiorly as well as septum cartilage.

Note that the inferior nasal concha is a bone in itself whereas the superior and middle nasal concha arise from the ethmoid bone.

The concha increases the surface area of the cavity which means air can be warmed and humidified before passing to the lungs.

23 The paranasal sinuses and the mastoid air cells

Paranasal sinuses

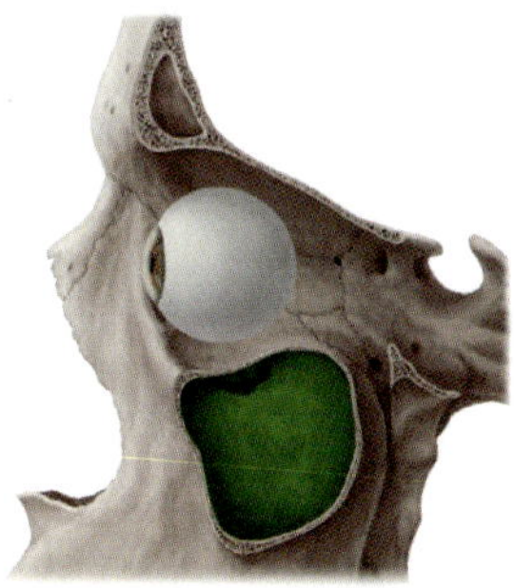

Fig 6.33 The maxillary sinus.

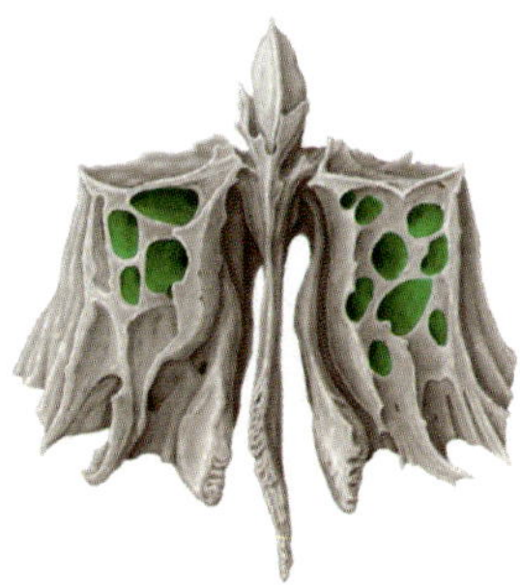

Fig 6.34 The ethmoid air cells.

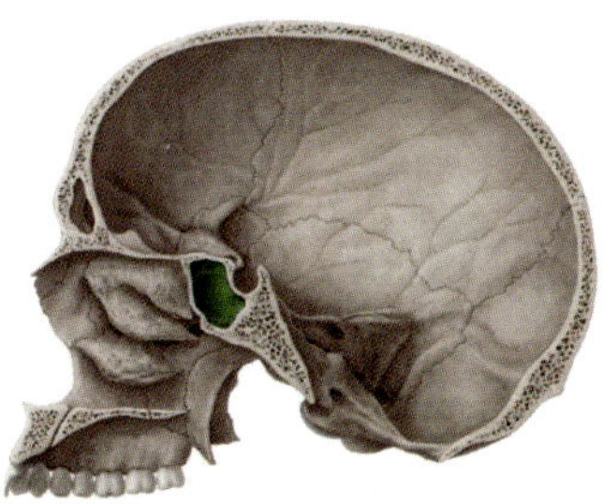

Fig 6.35 The sphenoid sinus.

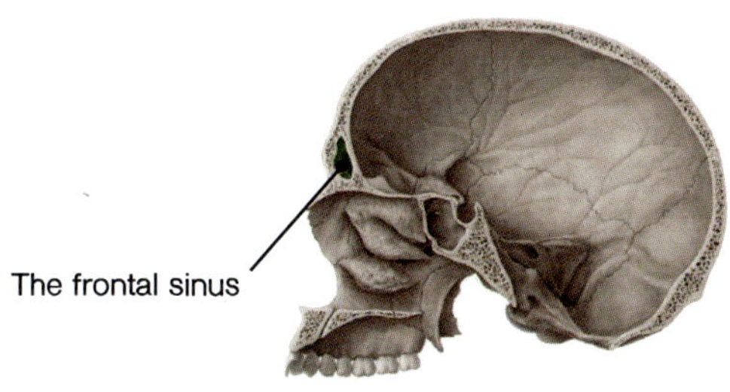

Fig 6.36 The frontal sinus.

'Paranasal' means surrounding the nose – they are positioned and named relative to the bone they are found in.

The mastoid bone is post-auricular and is where the mastoid air cells are found.

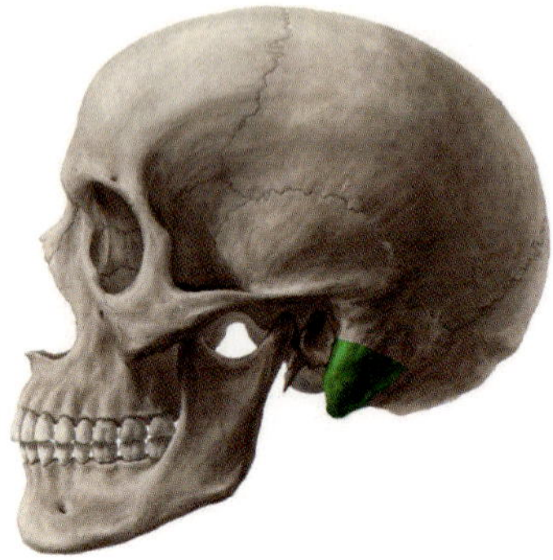

Fig 6.37 The mastoid process.

24 Surface landmarks for epidural injections

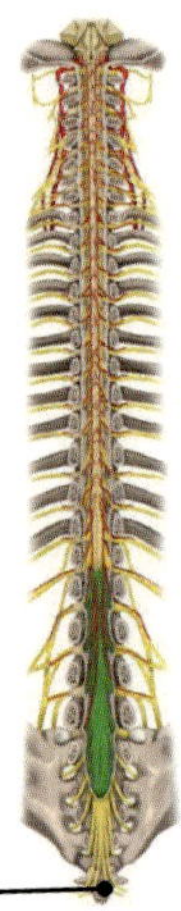

Fig 6.38 The spinal cord.

The spinal cord ends at L1/L2 in adults, and the nerves continue down individually (couda equinae). The nerves in the corda equinae will displace upon injection and reduce the risk of damage. The L3/L4 or L4/L5 junction can be used for these injections (L4 can be found medially from the superior iliac crests). Remember the level of L4 is the line that joins between the superior aspects of the iliac crests.
In children, sacral injections are used into the sacral foramina since the spinal cord isn't fully developed.

Good Medical Practice

Epidural space is outside of the dura mater – note that it does not contain any CSF; this is found in the subarachnoid space.

Subarachnoid injections are frequently used for anaesthesia, whereas epidurals are often for analgesia.[55]

25 Identify structures on a typical vertebra

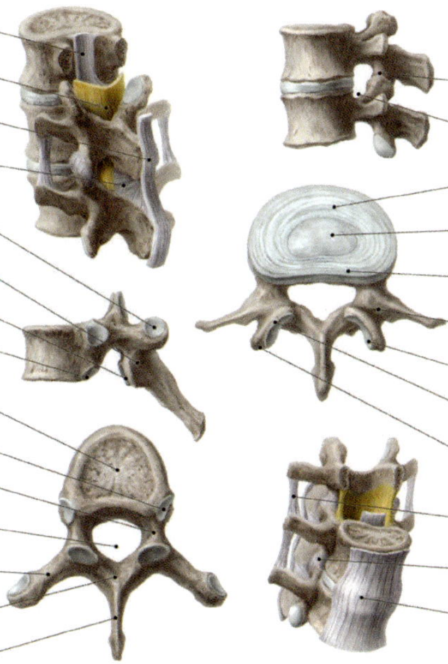

Fig 6.39 Thoracic and lumbar spines.

Good Medical Practice

The pedicle connects the body of the vertebra to the arch; the lamina connect the vertebra's processes (the spinous process with the transverse processes). No matter how bad my drawing is, I always try to make at least one sketch of bones I struggled with and labelled them from memory. Getting used to labelling and re-calling bones from memory was the best way for me to learn osteological specimens – plus it made learning them a little more fun, since learning bones can be very dull indeed.

26 The range of motions of different regions of the vertebral column

Flexion/Extension (bending forwards and backwards)[33]

- Cervix C1-C7 = large range of motion
- Upper ThoraxT1-T7 = no range of motion
- Lower ThoraxT7-T12 = very limited range of motion
- Lumbo-sacrum L1-S4 = large range of motion

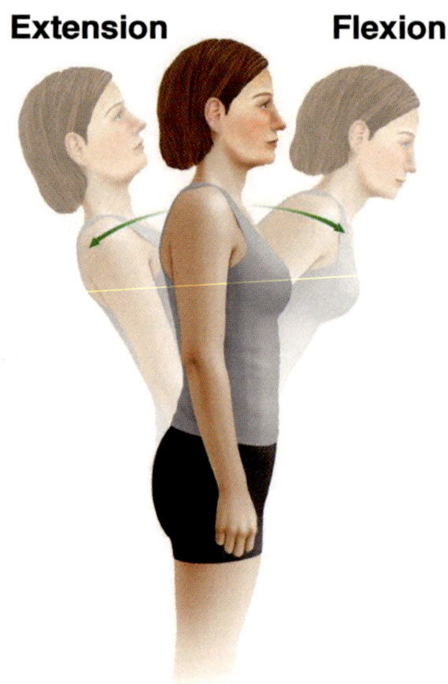

Fig 6.40 Flexion and extension of the spine.

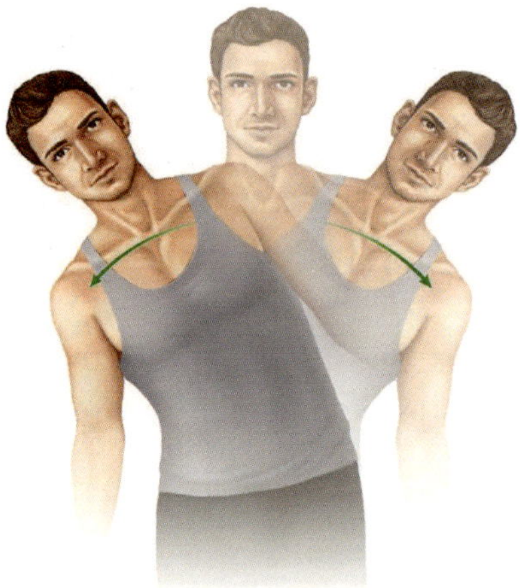

Fig 6.41 Lateral flexion of the spine.

Lateral flexion (bending side to side)[33]

- Cervix C1-C7 = large range of motion
- Upper Thorax T1-T7 = limited range of motion
- Lower Thorax T7-T12 = large range of motion
- Lumbo-sacrum L1-S4 = limited range of motion

Rotation[33]

- Cervix C1-C7 = large range of motion
- Upper Thorax T1-T7 = very limited range of motion
- Lower Thorax T7-T12 = large range of motion
- Lumbo-sacrum L1-S4 = no range of motion

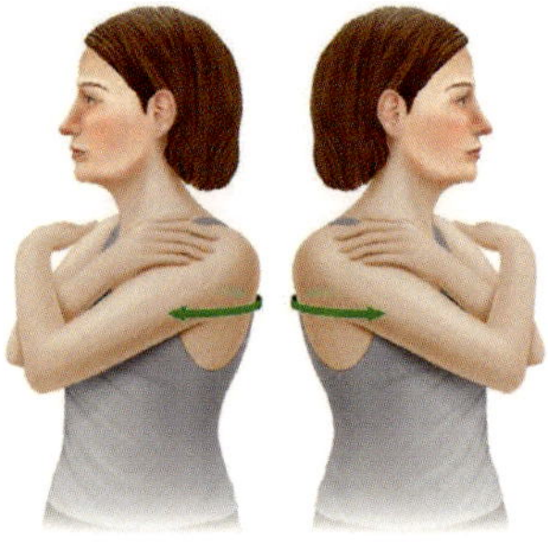

Fig 6.42 Rotation of the spine.

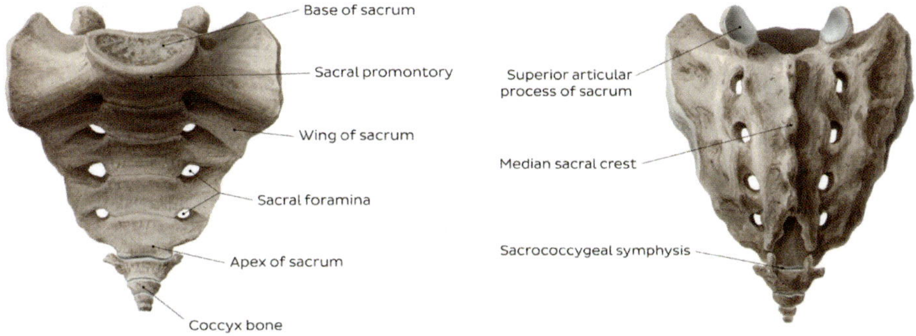

Fig 6.43 The sacrum and the coccyx.

Anatomical explanation of each region's range of movement:

Cervix – the atlanto-occipital joint and atlanto-axial joint allow full range of motion.

Upper Thorax – movement is restricted by the ribs and flexion/extension is prevented due to the long articular processes of the vertebra which prevent the vertebrae pivoting on one another.

Lower Thorax – here the ribs are 'floating', and therefore restrict movement less.

Lumbo-sacrum – vertebral processes are optimised for flexion and extension, and the articulations with each vertebra prevent rotation since they're vertical

27 Movements at the atlanto-occipital (AOJ) and atlanto-axial (AAJ) joints

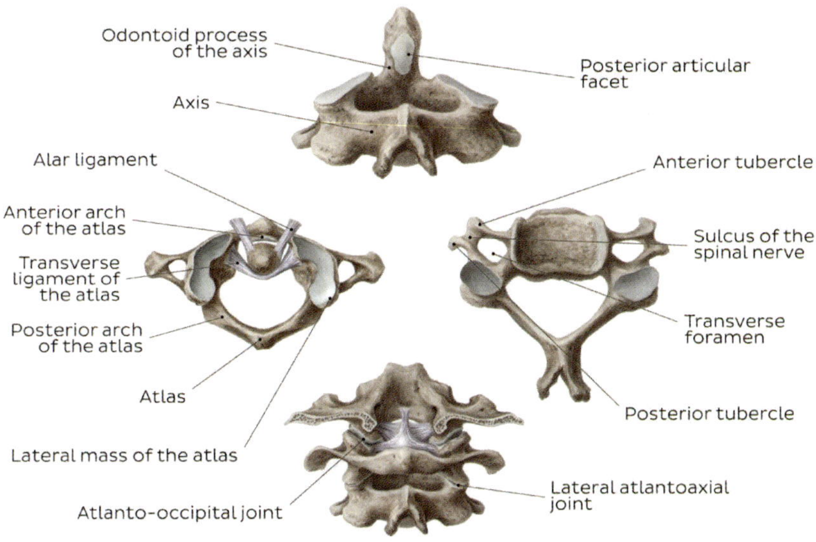

Fig 6.44 The atlas and axis.

Atlanto-Occipital Joint - The atlas (C1) forms a special joint type with the occipital bone; The superior articular surfaces of C1 articulate with the occipital condyles. This joint is responsible for flexion and extension of the head at the neck (nodding up and down – "*yes*").

Atlanto-Axial Joint - The axis (C2) forms a special joint with the atlas. The axis has a protruding part called the dens, also known as the dontoid process, which articulates with the anterior arch of the atlas. It is responsible for lateral rotation of the head around the neck (rotating the head side to side – "*no*").

Good Medical Practice

This is a skill so often required in your clinical studies and in your foundation I like to remember AOJ as "a ohh j"... 'ohh' as in 'yes', like you're nodding in agreement. Then remember that AAJ is the opposite

Final Remarks

So, this seems like a heck of a lot of information to not only learn, but to put into practice for the OSPE. I've structured the chapter by focusing more on the nerve examinations over the surface anatomy and the locations of bones. This is because the CN examinations are where your HNS practice should be largely focused on. Using this OSPE guidebook, along with other anatomy textbooks and Kenhub (which I personally recommend over any textbook), is sufficient for learning gross anatomy, but you really must practice performing the tests and examinations. Since the anatomy is going to be tested in the written exams, the OSPE is really where the actual practical tests are found.

Most importantly when practicing, it's good to get things wrong, it's good to forget things, and it's good to struggle initially to get the right order. We learn by making these mistakes – and you'll always remember to do it right next time if your colleague has made you aware of your mistakes. I initially kept forgetting to test the hypoglossal nerve with tongue protraction, but once other students pointed this out to me, I remember it better than the rest of the CN. Finally, in terms of remembering things, I firmly believe in testing yourself and active recall. Read through one of the LOs, try to then write it out from memory or run through it aloud in your room. You'll see how actively recalling information helps you learn, and actually remember information so much quicker than just passively reading these chapters.

I wish each and every student the best of luck with the OSPE, and I believe that wi
th practice and this book, you'll all do very well. Mastering the OSPE will be hugely helpful when you enter hospital placements, and you'll feel so much more confident when asked to examine patients as these techniques will come much more naturally to you, more so than in students from other medical schools where they don't have pre-clinical clinical assessments. Best of luck, Samuel Hammond

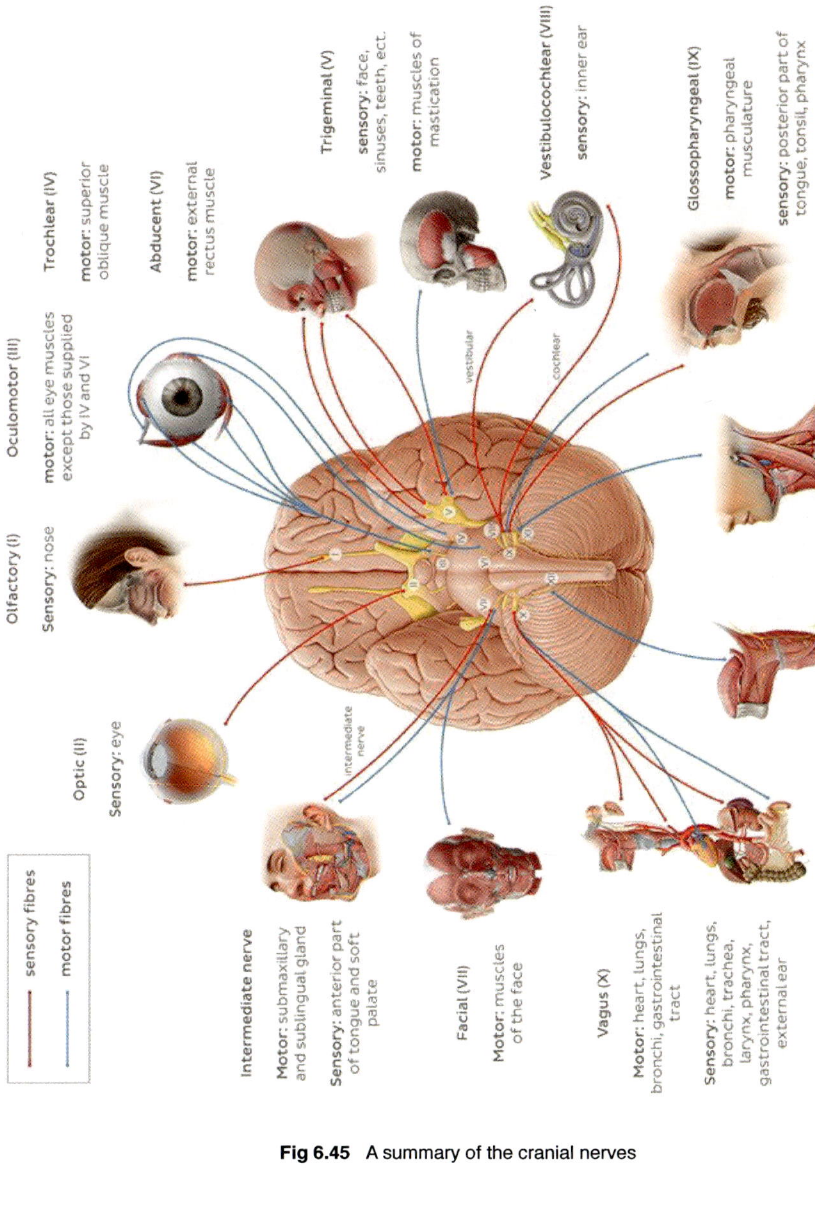

Fig 6.45 A summary of the cranial nerves

The Anatomy and Examinations of the Upper Limb

By Robert Vardanyan

Introduction to the chapter

Being the editor of this book, I've had the pleasure of reading every other author's work and refamiliarising myself with all the stations in the OSPE. And while difficulty in each OSPE station is a subjective matter, I can, without a doubt, confirm that the limbs stations are the hardest and most notorious. However, I wouldn't go so far as to say that they're the most clinically relevant in medical school, but in terms of difficulty, I think that the majority of students that have undertaken the OSPE would agree with me. There's just a ton more information to remember, a larger selection of questions that can come up, and you don't even know which limb station it is until you're reading the sheet right before the exam.

However, that's not to say that this station can't be made straightforward; you just need a solid understanding of limb anatomy. In fact, both stations (and everything in life really) can be made much more simple through mental organisation and grouping, and this is how I've structured the two limb chapters. We will discuss the anatomy and testing of the muscles, bones and joints first, then the nervous innervation, arterial supply, venous drainage, and lastly, the relevant anatomical structures. In fact, I have further divided both chapters based on anatomical regions, and it seems that the more distally you progress in the limb, the less you need to know about each muscle.

However, this is not the case for your pre-clinical anatomy studies outside of the OSPE. Whilst I hope that this book and this chapter will be a good resource when learning limb anatomy, it should not be the go-to guide or the anatomical atlas on which you base your studies. In fact, this was the biggest dilemma that arose when writing the limb chapters; how to make it concise OSPE guides and not anatomy textbook chapters, yet to cover all the bones, all the joints, and most muscles, nerves, veins, and arteries of the upper and lower limbs in sufficient detail. Therefore, for the sake of brevity, I sacrificed a lot of the 'Good Medical Practice' sections in these chapters.

I must, nonetheless, apologise for the immense amount of anatomy in this chapter and the next, as there can really be no shying away from the fact that a good understanding of the limb anatomy is required to excel in these stations. For my own peace of mind, I have decided to include all the anatomy detail required and can potentially be asked upon in subsequent follow-up questions, and that way I pass the responsibility on to you; whether you decide to learn and remember everything which I have written is your choice, but I have made it easier by highlighting the vital muscles with an asterisk.

Also, remember that when testing muscles or nerves, always apply resistance to the patient's movements whilst stabilising the joint upon which the muscle of interest is acting upon. This is usually done by stabilising the region/bones immediately proximal to the joint (such as the forearm when testing muscles that work on the wrist joint, or the proximal phalanx when assessing the FDS which flexes the proximal interphalangeal joints).[56]

Although, for the muscles acting upon the shoulder joint, stabilisation is not required – or rather, is difficult to perform and beyond the level of the OSPE – and so the muscle contractions should instead be palpated.[56] Examples of this are provided in the testing of the muscles of the anterior pectoral girdle and the intrinsic/extrinsic shoulder muscles, and palpation is not required for muscles that act distally to the shoulder joint. Also note that when testing the integrity of joints, no palpation or resistance should be applied to the patient's movements. Simply ask the patient (or better yet, demonstrate to the patient) to perform a specific movement while you observe.

In fact, it always good practice to demonstrate to the patient the movement you are asking them to perform, as it ensures clarity in communication and makes the encounter smoother.
Finally, note that when we discuss the 'arm' or 'upper arm', we are referring to the area between the shoulder and elbow, and not the upper limb as a whole.

Clinical Communication

"I have been asked to perform an examination of your arms and hands, and this involves me asking you to do various movement with them while I have a feel of your muscles and joints. I may also have to test your reflexes using a tendon hammer and the sensation on your skin using cotton wool. Would that be ok with you? Are you in any pain before we begin?"

1 Identify the bones and joints of the upper limb

From proximal to distal, we begin with the clavicle. The clavicle (known as the collarbone in lay terms) functions as the bridge between the shoulder girdle and the main trunk of the body. It's connection with the manubrium of the sternum, known as the **sternoclavicular joint**, forms the only bony articulation between the upper limb and the rest of the axial skeleton. As a result, the reinforcement of this synovial joint with numerous ligaments to ensure stability results in the sacrifice of a wide range of motion, although this means that sternoclavicular joint dislocation is rather rare.[57]

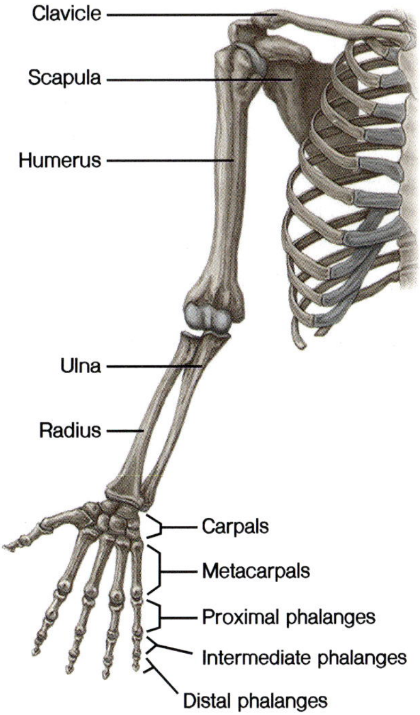

Fig 7.1 The bones of the upper limb.

Laterally, the scapula is a flat bone which forms the connection between the clavicle and the arm. The **acromioclavicular joint** is also a synovial joint, forming the articulation between acromion of the scapula and the lateral aspect of the clavicle. It is supported and stabilised through the **acromioclavicular**, **conoid**, and **trapezoid ligaments** (the latter two form the very strong **coracoclavicular** ligament, as labelled in **Fig 7.4**).

The scapula also makes an articulation with the posterior aspect of the thoracic wall, known as the **scapulo-thoracic joint**. This is something which you are required to know about in significant detail for your pre-clinical anatomy studies, but for the OSPEs, you can get away with just knowing the range of motions and testing of this joint, which in fact is not a true synovial joint or an anatomical joint. The scapulo-thoracic joint is involved in the protraction, retraction, rotation, elevation, and depression of the upper limb through the movements of the scapula across the ribcage.

Elevation of the scapula results in the 'shrugging of shoulders' motion, whereas depression results in a movement similar to slouching. Protraction is the when the scapula moves anteriorly and laterally. Retraction is when the scapula moves posteriorly and medially. Medial rotation of the scapula results in the medial rotation of the upper limb (from the arm), and lateral rotation of the scapula results in the lateral rotation of the upper limb.

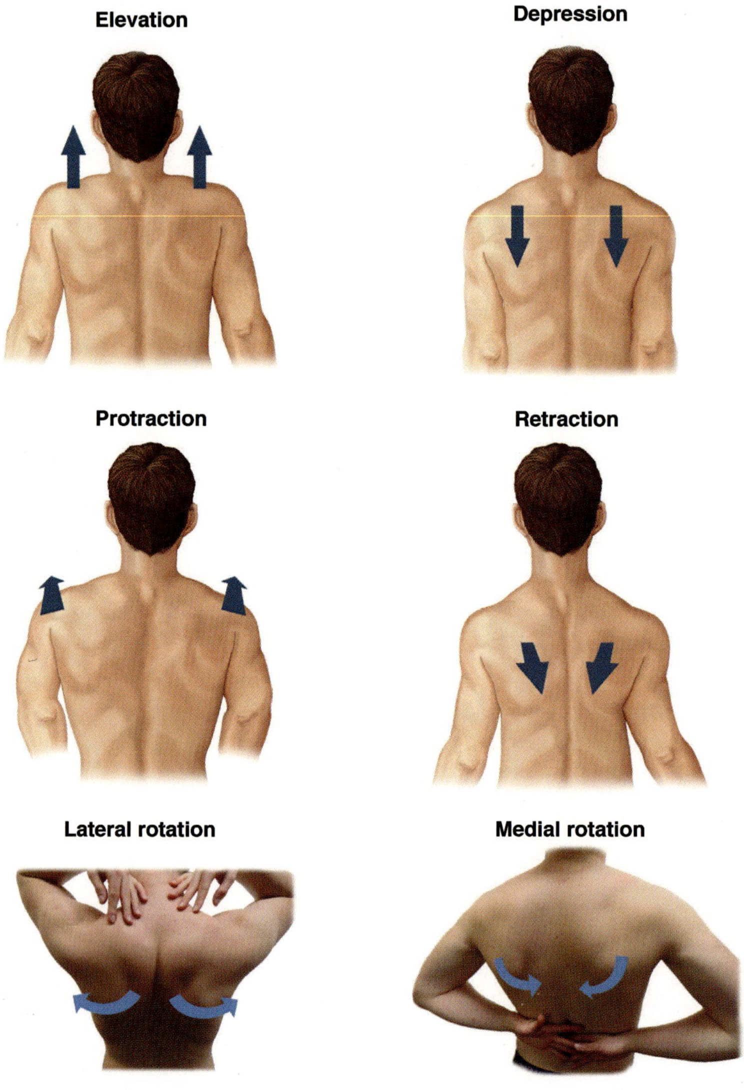

Fig 7.2 The motions of the scapulo-thoracic joint

Finally, the last joint of the shoulder girdle is the **glenohumeral** (shoulder) **joint**. This ball and socket synovial joint is formed through the articulation of the head of the humerus and the glenoid cavity, and it is one of the most highly mobile joints in the body, with the upper arm having a significantly wide range of motion about the centre point of the humeral head. However, this is at the cost of joint stability, regardless of the numerous ligaments, the surrounding joint capsule, or the plethora of muscles that attach to or bind around the joint to assist in mobility.[58]

Fig 7.3 The seven motions of the glenohumeral joint.

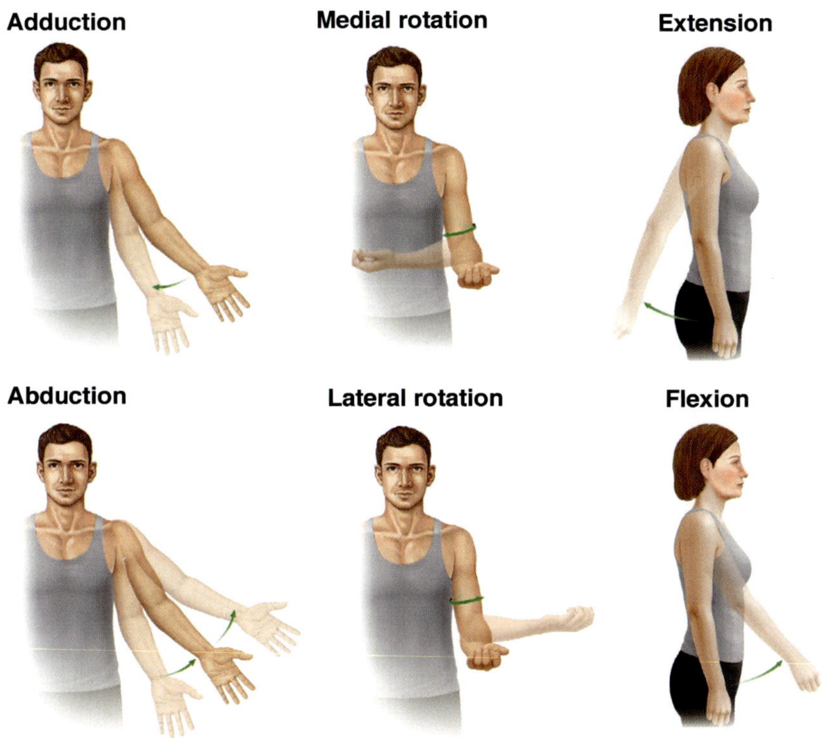

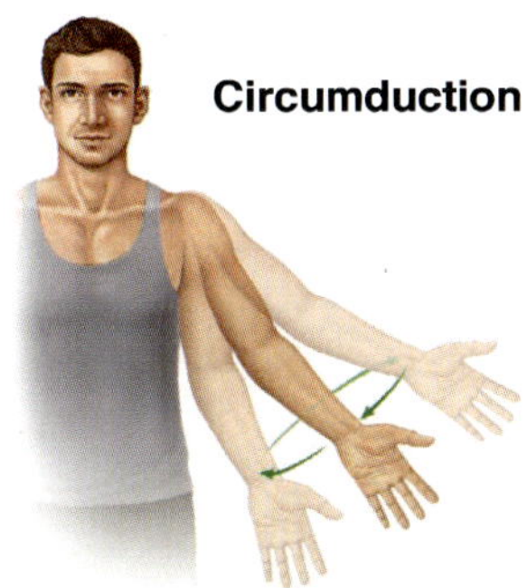

Extra medical notes

As mentioned, the mobility of the glenohumeral joint is at the expense of stability, so shoulder dislocation is common. This is when the humeral head slips out of the glenoid cavity of the scapula, and it is treated non-surgically through a procedure known as shoulder reduction.[59]

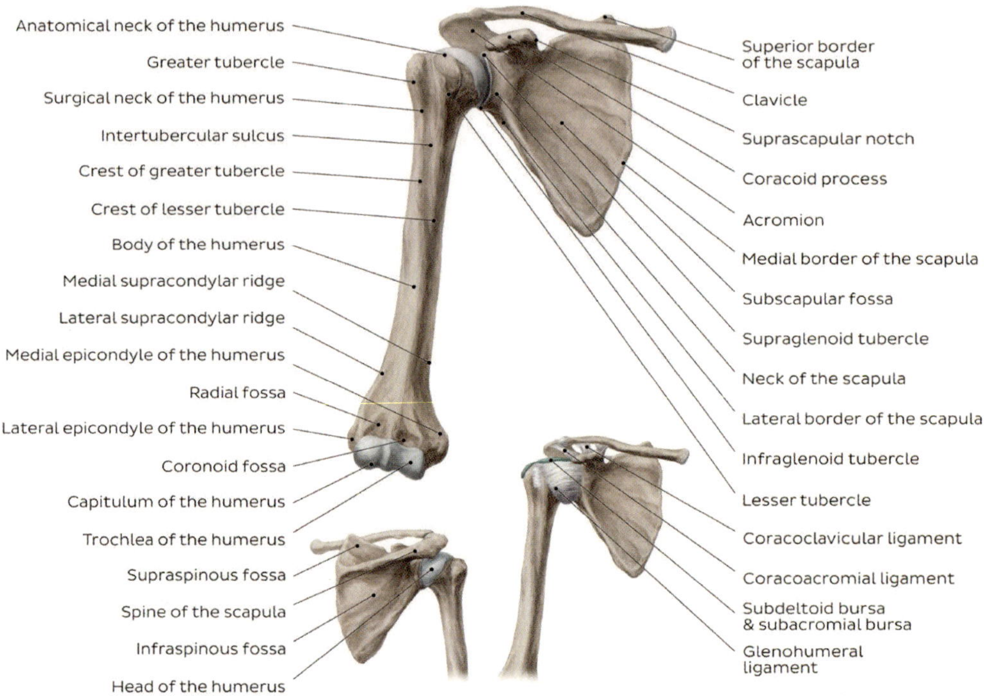

Fig 7.4 The ligaments, bones, and respective surface landmarks of the shoulder girdle and upper arm.

The upper arm is formed upon the humerus, a long bone which articulates with the shoulder girdle (through the glenohumeral joint) and the forearm (through the elbow joint). I must stress that every labelled aspect in **Fig 7.4** is required knowledge for your pre-clinical anatomy curriculum and it forms a large part of the foundations to the upper limb station in the OSPE. Note also the surgical neck of the humerus, which is a location with a tendency to fracture.

The elbow joint is a synovial hinge joint, permitting motion in only one plane. It is an articulation of the humerus with the radius and the ulna bones of the forearm. The **trochlea** of the humerus articulates with the **trochlear notch** (formed by the olecranon and coronoid process) of the ulna, and the **capitulum** of the humerus articulates with the **head of the radius**.

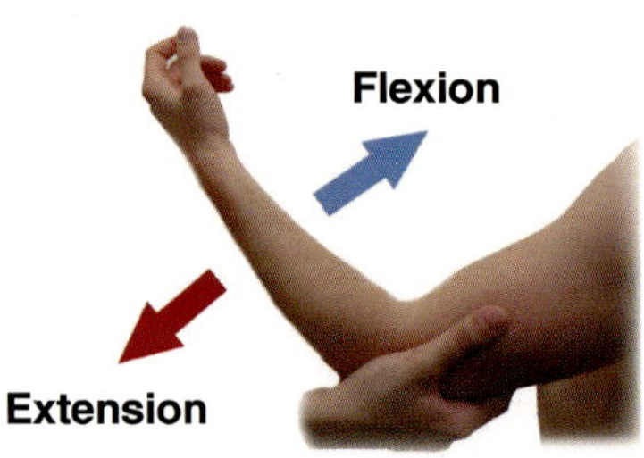

Therefore, the elbow can only undergo flexion or extension. You should not confuse pronation/supination of the radio-ulnar joints or medial/lateral rotation of the humerus at the glenohumeral joint as being a motion of the elbow, which many students do.

Fig 7.5 Flexion and extension of the elbow joint while it is being stabilised.

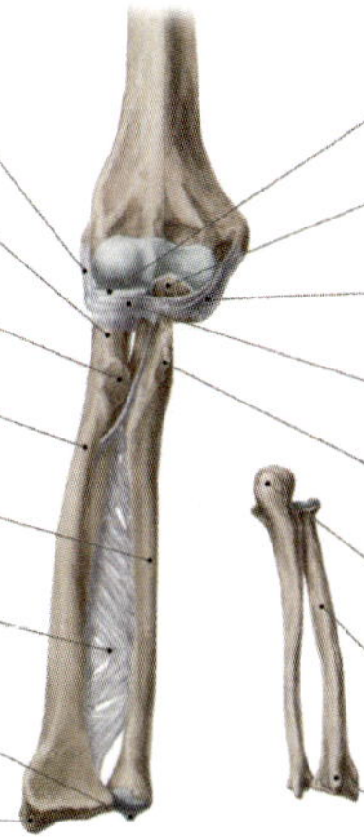

Fig 7.6 The elbow joint and the bones of the forearm; the radius and ulna.

The radius and ulna are the two bones of the forearm, and articulate with one another at the **proximal and distal radio-ulnar joints**. At the distal radio-ulnar joint, the radius is able to pivot around the ulna to produce the **pronation** and **supination** movements of the forearm.

Learning notes

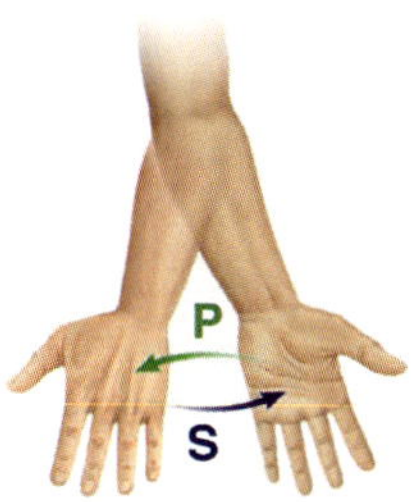

Fig 7.7 Pronation and supination of the forearm through the pivoting of the radius around the distal radio-ulnar joint, and to a much lesser extent, the proximal radio-ulnar joint. 'P' and 'S' represent pronation and supination.

Pronation is turning your palm towards the **p**avement, while **s**upination is turning your palm to **s**ky.
Another way to remember this is:
Pronation - **'P'** - playing basketball.
Supination - **'S'** - soup bowl.

The proximal radio-ulnar joint is formed by the head of the radius and the radial notch of the ulna, and it is not a part of the elbow joint but it shares the same articular capsule.

The distal radio-ulnar joint is formed by the articulation of the head of the ulna and the ulnar notch of the radius. It contains an **articular disk** which stabilises the distal radio-ulnar joint when the radius pivots around the ulna and it separates the distal radio-ulnar joint from the wrist joint.

The wrist joint is a condyloid connection of the forearm and the hand. It is formed by the articulation of the distal end of the radius, the articular disk, and three of the proximal carpal bones (**scaphoid, lunate, triquetrum**). The ulna is not part of the wrist joint; it is separated by the articular disk, and only articulates with the ulnar notch of the radius distally.[33]
For this reason, the wrist joint is known as the **radiocarpal joint.**

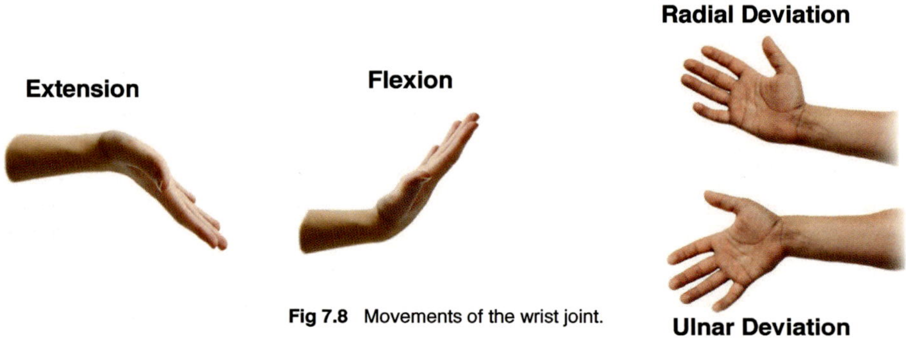

Fig 7.8 Movements of the wrist joint.

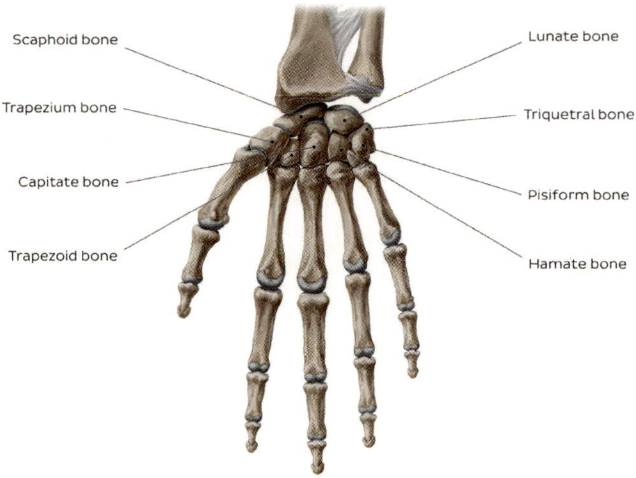

Fig 7.9 The carpal bones of the hand.

The eight carpal bones are arranged in two rows and form the most proximal bones of the hand. Small and irregularly shaped, the carpal bones together form a convex surface that articulates with the radius at the wrist joint and a concave arch which forms the floor of the carpal tunnel.

Note that the **pisiform is a sesamoid bone** (embedded in the tendon of the flexor carpi ulnaris) that does not take part in the formation of the wrist joint.

Key learning notes

The names of the carpal bones are, from the lateral to medial:
1st (proximal) row: scaphoid, lunate, triquetrum, pisiform
2nd (distal) row: trapezium, trapezoid, capitate, and hamate.

The **carpal tunnel** is a narrow canal found on the palmar side of the hand where the four tendons of the **flexor digitorum profundus**, four tendons of the **flexor digitorum superficialis**, the tendon of the **flexor pollicis longus**, and the **median nerve** pass through from the forearm into the hand. The tunnel is formed by the carpal bones and a strong fibrous band, known as the **flexor retinaculum**, which arches over them. The flexor retinaculum attaches to the scaphoid and trapezium bones on the radial side, and the pisiform and the hook of Hamate on the ulnar side of the hand. This is also discussed later on in ***LO 6***, regarding the relevant upper limb structures. A common medical condition of note is carpal tunnel syndrome (CTS), which arises when one or more of the nine flexor tendons swells and further narrows the canal, resulting in the entrapment and compression of the median nerve.

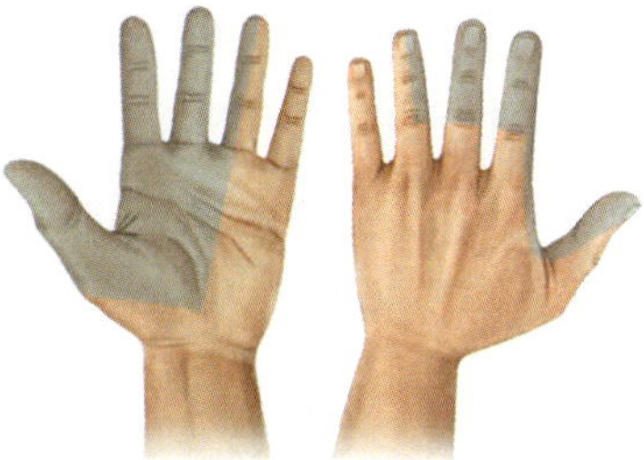

Fig 7.10 The location of hand pain in CTS as a result of median nerve compression.

With regards to memorising the positioning of the carpal bones, a good mnemonic is always useful. For example, **'Straight Line To Pinky, Here Comes The Thumb'** is a mnemonic to remember the carpal bones in a circular order starting from the scaphoid, progressing towards the pisiform near the fifth digit (pinky), and then returning to the trapezium bone near the first digit (thumb). There are plenty of other mnemonics out there, but some learners try practicing things they can't handle.

There are five metacarpals, five proximal phalanges, four intermediate phalanges, and five distal phalanges in each hand. Alongside the carpal bones, this sums up to 27 bones per hand.

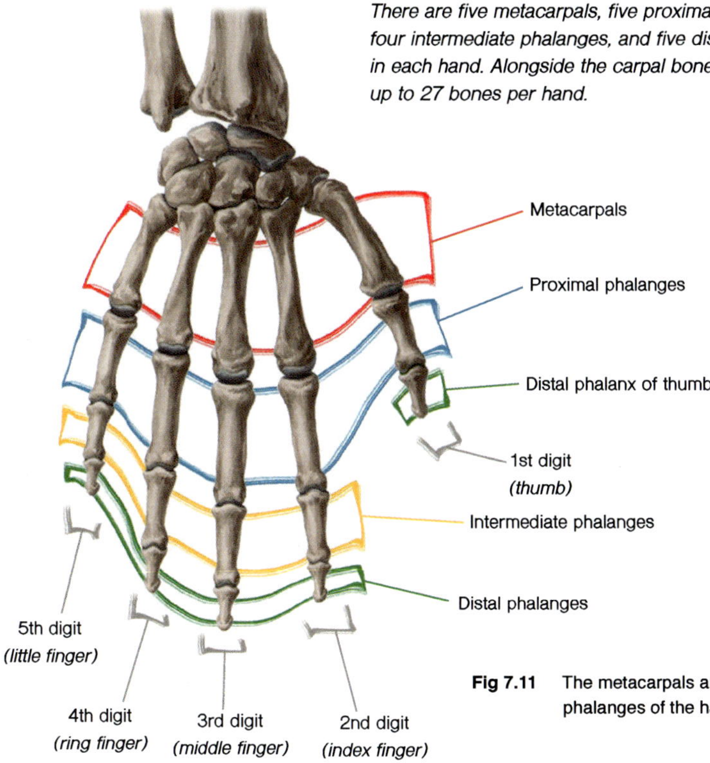

Fig 7.11 The metacarpals and phalanges of the hand.

The metacarpals are long bones within the hand that connect the phalanges (bones of the fingers and toes) to the carpal bones in the hand. Flexion of the **metacarpophalangeal joints** brings about the protrusion of the knuckles. Although limited, they can also **extend**, **adduct**, **abduct**, and **circumduct**.

Note that the **thumb only has proximal and distal phalanges**, and lacks an intermediate phalanx. This is unlike the other four digits of the hand, which have all three bone types, but similar to the big toe (hallux).

2 The muscles of the upper limb

The muscles that act upon the upper limb are numerous in number and diverse in function. Therefore, we will discuss the muscles by categorising them into nine different groups based upon anatomical location. These groups are:

1) Anterior chest wall
2) Extrinsic shoulder muscles
3) Intrinsic shoulder muscles
4) Anterior muscles of the upper arm
5) Posterior muscles of the upper arm
6) Anterior muscles of forearm
7) Posterior muscles of forearm
8) Intrinsic muscles of the hand

Within each of these groups we will discuss the functions of the muscles, relevant tendons and joints, the appropriate clinical examinations, and brief neurovasculature. Please keep in mind that neurovasculature will be appropriately explored in later learning objectives. Furthermore, we will delve deeper into only some of the muscles listed, as this is what is required within the OSPEs. **These key muscles will be marked with an asterisk**.

1) The anterior chest wall (pectoral girdle)

The key muscles of interest are the **pectoralis major** and the **serratus anterior**, but the pectoralis minor and subclavius will also be discussed.

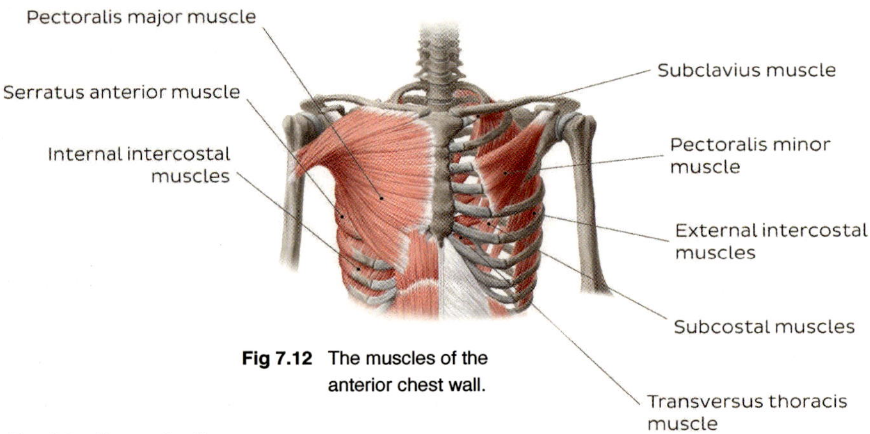

Fig 7.12 The muscles of the anterior chest wall.

Pectoralis major*

The pectoralis major is a large, fan-shaped, superficial muscle, which makes up most of the chest wall. It **adducts, flexes, and medially rotates the humerus** (and therefore the upper limb), and it arises from the **medial half of the clavicle**, the **superior sixth costal cartilages**, and the **aponeurosis of the external oblique** muscle. It inserts into the **lateral lip of the intertubercular sulcus**, and it is innervated by the **medial and lateral pectoral nerve**.

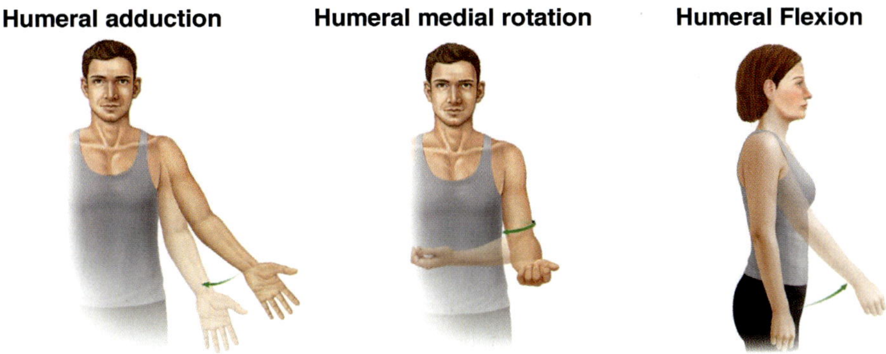

Fig 7.13 The movements of the upper limb caused by the action of pectoralis major.

To test the pectoralis major muscle, ask the patient to **adduct their arm** while their elbow is flexed, against resistance. This is similar to the wings of a chicken, and you can use this comparison to verbally clarify what you want the patient to do. As the examiner, you must **feel** the action of the pectoralis major by placing your hand on their chest and by **resisting** the adduction of their upper arm. This is the easy one of the three common tests.

You can also assess the function of the pectoralis major by asking the patient to medially rotate their arm (flexed at the elbow), whilst you provide **resistance** and **palpate** their pectoralis major. This is pictured in **Fig 7.14**.

To request this test from the patient ask them to: *"Bend your elbows and try to move your forearm into your centre, while I apply resistance and feel your chest?"*

Lastly, you can ask the patient to flex their arm whilst you resist the rise of their upper limb and palpate the pectoralis major.

These are also three of the tests that you can conduct to assess the **glenohumeral joint**. However, no resistance to motion or palpation of muscles is required when testing joint function.

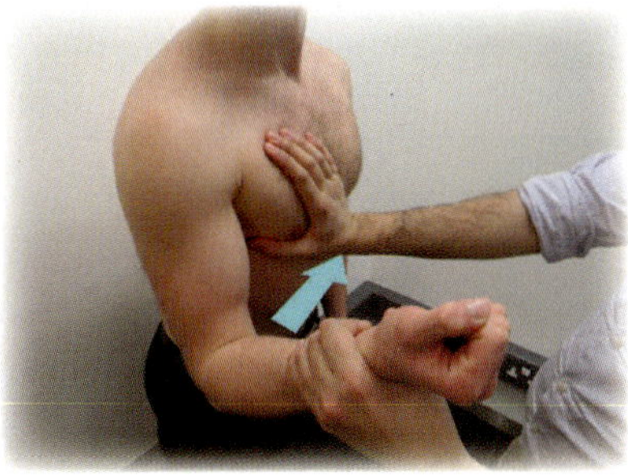

Fig 7.14 Testing the pectoralis major through medial rotation of the upper arm.

Pectoralis minor

The pectoralis minor lies deep to the pectoralis major, and it is innervated by the **medial pectoral nerve**. It's function is to **stabilise the scapula** by drawing it anteroinferiorly against the thoracic wall, and it originates from the anterior surface of **ribs III - V** and inserts into the **coracoid process** of the scapula.

Subclavius

The subclavius arises from the **first costochondral joint**, and it inserts into the **middle third of the clavicle**. It's function is to **stabilise and depress the clavicle** (and therefore the pectoral girdle).

Serratus Anterior*

The serratus anterior arises from the **lateral aspects of ribs I - VIII** and it inserts into the **medial border of the scapula** (refer to **Fig 7.4**). This allows it to **laterally rotate the scapula** and **protracts the scapula against the ribcage**. It is innervated by the **long thoracic nerve**, which if damaged, no longer allows the serratus anterior to hold the scapula in a protracted state against the ribcage and allows it to protrude, leading to the 'winged scapula'.

To test the serratus anterior muscle, ask the patient to push their arm out whilst you, as the examiner, feel the action of the serratus anterior by placing your hand on the posteriolateral aspect of their chest and by resisting the protraction of their scapula by resisting them pushing their arm out. This is pictured in **Fig 7.15**.

To request this test from the patient ask:
"Can you push your arm out as far as you can whilst I resist you and feel under your arm."

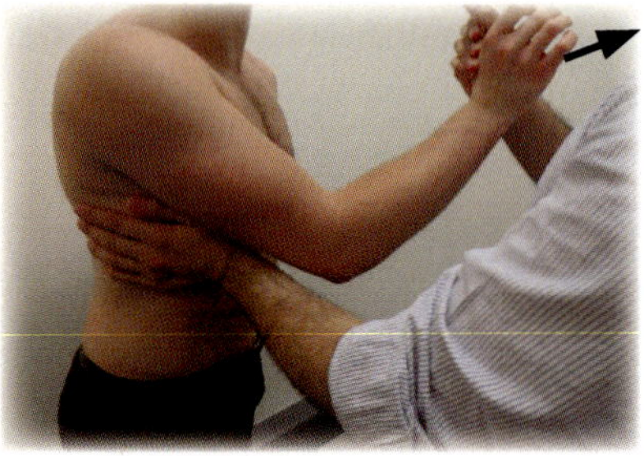

Fig 7.15 Testing the serratus anterior through the protraction of the scapula.

2) The extrinsic shoulder muscles

These muscles originate from the trunk wall and insert into the bones of the shoulder girdle, specifically the scapula, clavicle, and humerus. The key muscles of interest are the superficial extrinsic shoulder muscles - the **latissimus dorsi** and **trapezius muscles**. However, we will also briefly discuss the deep extrinsic shoulder muscles - the rhomboids and the levator scapulae.

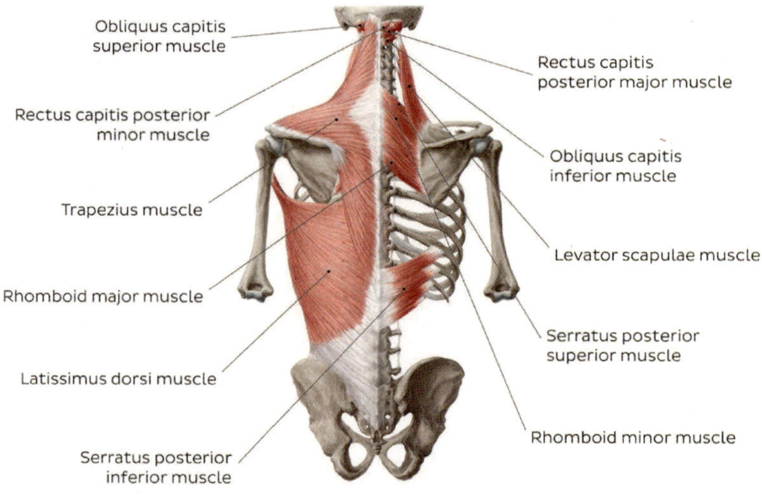

Fig 7.16 The muscles of the posterior chest wall.

Latissimus dorsi*

The latissimus dorsi is a large flat muscle that twists upon itself to insert into the **intertubercular groove** of the humerus, between the insertion point of the pectoralis major (lateral lip of intertubercular sulcus) and the teres major (medial lip of intertubercular sulcus). It originates from the **vertebrae T7–T12**, **iliac crest**, **ribs IX - XII**, and the inferior angle of the scapula. However, there is significant variation in origin of the latissimus dorsi amongst individuals.[60] Innervated by the **long scapular nerve**, it's functions are to **extend**, **adduct**, and **medially rotate the upper limb**.

Though not vital for the OSPEs, to test the latissimus dorsi muscle, you can do one of the tests relevant to the pectoralis major. Ask the patient to adduct their arm while their elbow is flexed, against resistance. As the examiner, you will be standing behind the patient in order to feel the action of the latissimus dorsi by placing your hand on their back and by resisting the adduction of their upper arm.
This is also a test that you can conduct to assess the **glenohumeral joint**. However, no resistance to motion or palpation of muscles is required when testing joints.

To request this test from the patient ask them:
"Can you stick your arm out like a chicken and then try to bring your elbows to your side while I try to resist you?"

Trazpezius*

The trapezius is a large muscle that is divided into three parts to reflect it's actions.
It is divided into (from superior to inferior) the **descending, transverse, and ascending trapezius**. It originates from the **occipital bone**, the **nuchal ligament**, and the **spinous processes of C7-T12**. It then inserts at the **clavicle**, **acromion**, and the **scapular spine** in order to **elevate and rotate** the scapula, **retract the scapula**, and **depress the scapula**

.

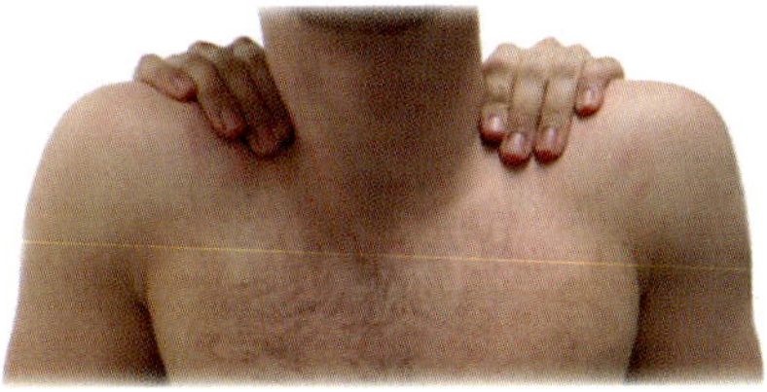

Fig 7.17 Testing the trapezius muscle by asking the patient to raise their shoulders against resistance.

It is innervated by CN XI, the **accessory nerve**.

To test the function of the trapezius muscle, ask the patient to raise their shoulder whilst you, as the examiner, resist this elevation.
This is pictured in **Fig 7.17**.

To request this test from the patient ask them to:
"Shrug your shoulders whilst I try to resist you."

Levator Scapulae

The levator scapulae is a small strap-like muscle that originates from the transverse processes of the C1-C4 vertebrae and attaches to the medial border of the scapula.
It is innervated by the dorsal scapular nerve and it helps in the **elevation of the scapula**.

Rhomboid major

It originates from the spinous processes of T2-T5 vertebrae and attaches to the medial border of the scapula. It is also inneravted by the dorsal scapular nerve and it **retracts** and **medially rotates the scapula**.

Rhomboid minor

Originating from the spinous processes of C7-T1 vertebrae, the rhomboid minor attaches to the medial border of the scapula and helps in it's **retraction** and **medial rotation**. It is also innervated by the dorsal scapular nerve.

3) The intrinsic shoulder muscles

These muscles originate from the scapula or clavicle and attach to the humerus.
The key muscles of interest are the **deltoid, teres major**, and **rotator cuff muscles**.

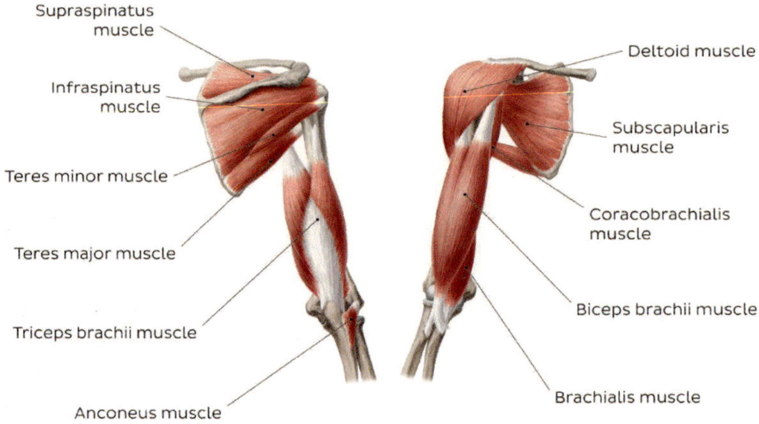

Fig 7.18 The intrinsic shoulder and upper arm muscles. The anconeus muscle pictured above is actually a part of the posterior compartment of the forearm.

Deltoid*

Originating from the **acromion, spine of the scapula, and lateral third of clavicle**, the deltoid is a prominent muscle and the main **abductor of the arm**.

In this regard, the deltoid is an antagonist of latissimus dorsi and pectoralis major.
It is innervated by the **axillary nerve** (like the teres minor and the long head of the triceps brachii), and it inserts into the **deltoid tuberosity** of the humerus.

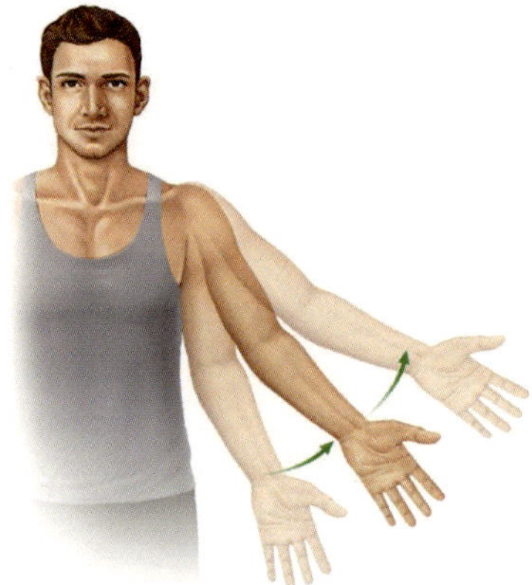

Fig 7.19 Upper limb abduction.

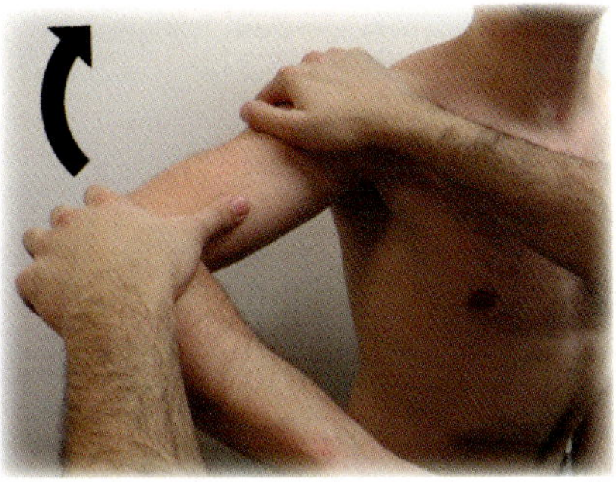

Fig 7.20 Testing the deltoid muscle through the abduction of the upper limb.

To test the function of the deltoid, ask the patient flex their elbow and **raise their arm** to their side, like a chicken. As they do this, you must gently resist the abduction of their arm and feel the action of the deltoid.
This is pictured in **Fig 7.20**.

To request this test from the patient ask them to: *"Bend your elbow and raise your arm up to your shoulder level whilst I try to resist you."*

It is also best to firstly show the patient the action you are asking them to perform.

Teres major

The teres major is a small muscle that originates from the **lateral aspect of the inferior angle of the scapula** and it inserts into the **medial lip of the intertubercular sulcus**.
As a way of remembering it's insertion, remember that the latissimus dorsi inserts between two 'majors' at the intertubercular sulcus (which is essentially a groove between the greater and lesser tubercles of the humerus).
The teres major functions to **adduct**, **retract**, and **medially rotate** the humerus, and it is innervated by the **lower subscapular nerve**. It therefore functions to assist the latissimus dorsi. Also, it is often confused as one of the rotator cuff muscles (of which there are four, including the teres minor), but fundamentally, it does not insert at a point to encapsulate the glenohumeral joint to stabilise it. Furthermore, testing of the teres major is shown and discussed in **Fig 7.22**.

Rotator cuff muscles*

There are four rotator cuff muscles, and like the teres major, they all originate from various points of the scapula. However, unlike the teres major, they all attach to the tubercles of the humerus to stabilise the glenohumeral joint amongst their other functions.

The **subscapularis** is the only rotator cuff muscle to originate anteriorly to the scapula, at **subscapular fossa**. It is also the only rotator cuff muscle to attach to the **lesser tubercle** of the humerus. It **medially rotates** the arm, and is innervated by the upper and lower subscapular nerves.

The **supraspinatous** originates from the **supraspinous fossa** of the scapula and is innervated by the suprascapular nerve. It then inserts at the **greater tubercle** of the humerus and it functions as the main **abductor of the humerus** for the first 15° and then continues to assist the deltoid in the rest of the arm abduction.

The **infraspinatous** originates from the **infraspinous fossa** of the scapula and is also innervated by the suprascapular nerve. It then inserts at the **greater tubercle** of the humerus and it functions to **laterally rotate** the arm.

The **teres minor** originates from the **lateral border** of the scapula, just superior to the teres major. It then inserts at the **greater tubercle** of the humerus and functions to **laterally rotate** the humerus. It is innervated by the **axillary nerve**, which also provides innervation to the deltoid and the long head of the triceps brachii.

Compound movements are used as a quick test for the shoulder joint and various rotator cuff muscles simultaneously.
Specifically, to assess **lateral rotation and abduction** together, ask the patient to put their hand behind their neck. This is whilst you, as the examiner, apply resistance to the arm and palpate the rotator cuff muscles.
The patient's movement is pictured in **Fig 7.21**.

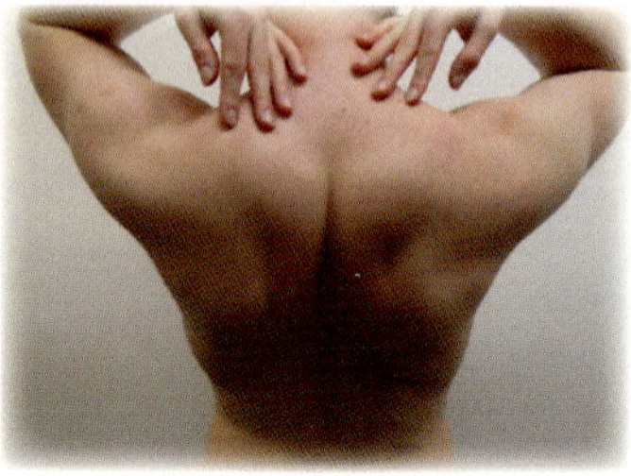

Fig 7.21 Testing the lateral rotation and abduction of the upper arm simultaneously.

If pathology is observed, then specific testing must be done for each muscle that was tested (the teres minor, supraspinatous, and infraspinatous), but for the OSPE, general screening for rotator cuff function is sufficient.

Furthermore, to assess the **medial rotation of the shoulder joint** and the subscapularis (alongside the teres major), ask the patient to put their hand as far up their back as possible. Again, this is whilst you, as the examiner, apply resistance to the arm and palpate the rotator cuff muscles.
The patient's movement is pictured in **Fig 7.22**.

It is best to firstly demonstrate the action you are asking them to perform.

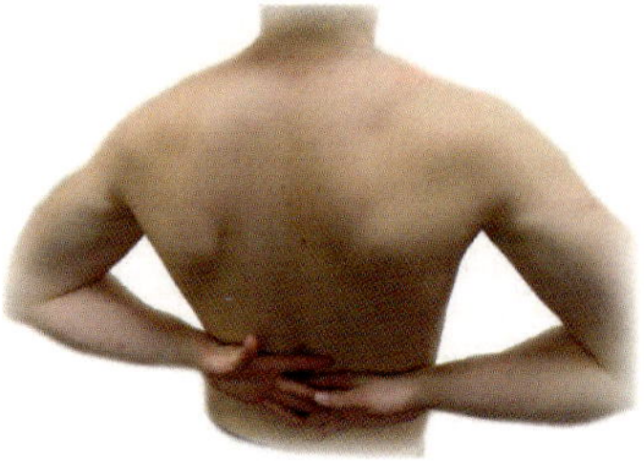

Fig 7.22 The test to assess both the teres major and the subscapularis through medial rotation, adduction, and retraction of the upper arm.

4) Anterior muscles of the arm

These three muscles are all located in the anterior compartment of the arm and are all innervated by the musculocutaneous nerve and mainly supplied by the brachial artery.
The muscles are the biceps brachii, brachialis, and coracobrachialis (pictured in **Fig 7.18**).

Biceps brachii*

The biceps brachii (meaning the two-headed muscle of the arm) is a superficial **flexor** and the main **supinator** of the forearm. It is found anteriorly to the humerus, but it actually has no attachment to the humerus, and it originates solely from the anterior aspects of the scapula. The short head originates from the **coracoid process of the scapula** and is found medially to the long head, which originates from the **supraglenoid tubercle** of the scapula and descends down the humerus through the **intertubercular groove** (enclosed by the **transverse humeral ligament**) to merge with the short head. Following this, the biceps brachii then attaches to the **radial tuberosity** and gives off an **aponeurosis** which joins the fascia of the forearm.

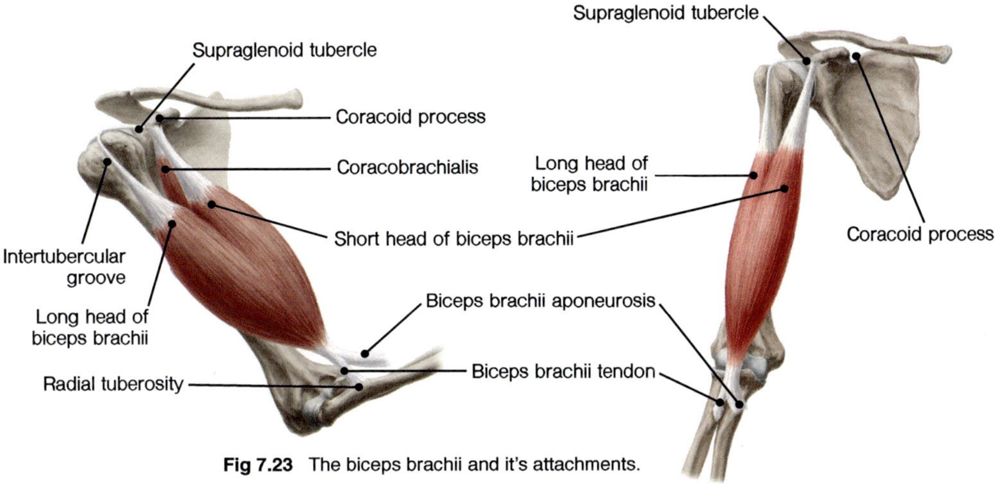

Fig 7.23 The biceps brachii and it's attachments.

To test the function of the biceps brachii, ask the patient to flex their elbow whilst you resist the movement. You must also stabilise the elbow joint during this examination.
This is pictured in **Fig 7.24**.

To request this test from the patient ask them to:
"Bend your elbow whilst I stabilise it and resist your movement by holding your forearm"

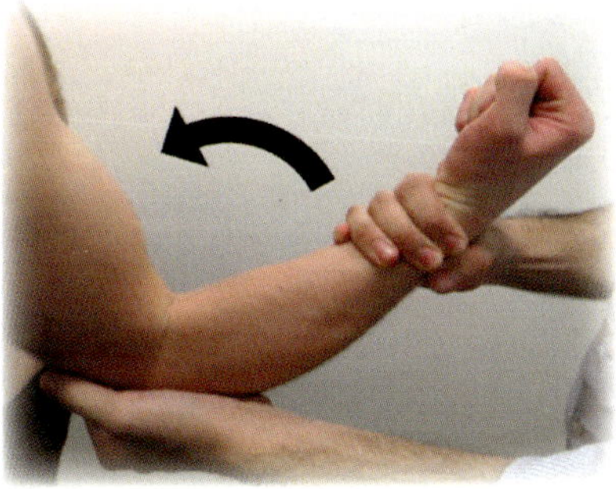

Fig 7.24 Testing the biceps brachii muscle through the flexion of the forearm.

Good Medical Practice

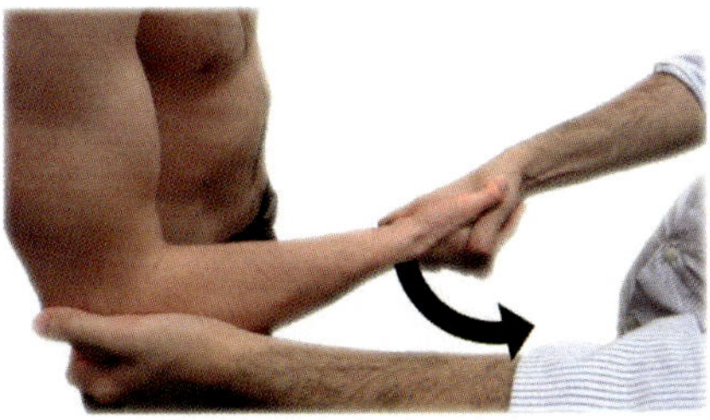

Fig 7.25 Testing the biceps brachii muscle through the supination of the forearm.

As the biceps brachii is also involved in the supination of the forearm, another test can also be performed to assess the function of the muscle. This involves stabilising the patients elbow joint and asking them to supinate their forearm (with their fist clenched) whilst you, as the examiner, resist this motion.

To request this test from the patient ask them to:
"Turn your wrist outwards whilst I apply some resistance against it and stabilise your elbow"

It is best to demonstrate this action first.

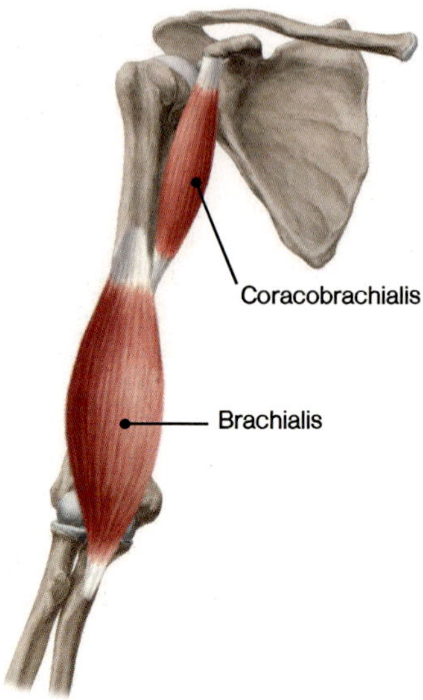

Fig 7.26 The brachialis and the coracobrachialis.

Brachialis

The brachialis has its origins near the middle of the humeral shaft and it attaches distally to ulnar tuberosity. It is deep to the biceps brachii and it is mainly innervated by the **musculocutaneous** nerve, but it also has some innervation from the radial nerve. Surprisingly, it is the main **flexor of the forearm** and it produces more power than the biceps brachii.[33,61] This is despite the biceps brachii being larger in size and spanning the entirety of the humerus. The brachialis also forms the floor of the cubital fossa.

Coracobrachialis

The coracobrachialis also lies deep to the biceps brachii, and it originates from the coracoid process of the scapula (like the short head of the biceps brachii and pectoralis minor).

The coracobrachialis assists in the flexion and adduction of the humerus, to which it attaches to at the middle of the medial aspect of. It is also innervated by the **musculocutaneous** nerve.[33,61]

5) Posterior muscles of the arm

The posterior compartment of the arm contains only one muscle, the triceps brachii (pictured in **Fig 7.18**).

Triceps brachii*

The triceps brachii comprises three heads that converge together to form a common tendon that inserts distally at the **olecranon of the ulna**. The long head originates from the **infraglenoid tubercle**, while the medial and lateral heads originate from the **posterior surface of the humerus**. The medial head originates inferiorly and the lateral head originates superiorly to the radial groove. With the lateral head considered to be the strongest, the triceps brachii works in the **extension of the forearm**, antagonising the muscles of the anterior compartment of the arm.[61] As the long head originates from the infraglenoid tubercle, it also has some function in adducting the arm. The triceps brachii is innervated by the **radial nerve**, and the triceps reflex is used to test its function.[33,61] This will be discussed in more detail in the reflexes section of LO3.

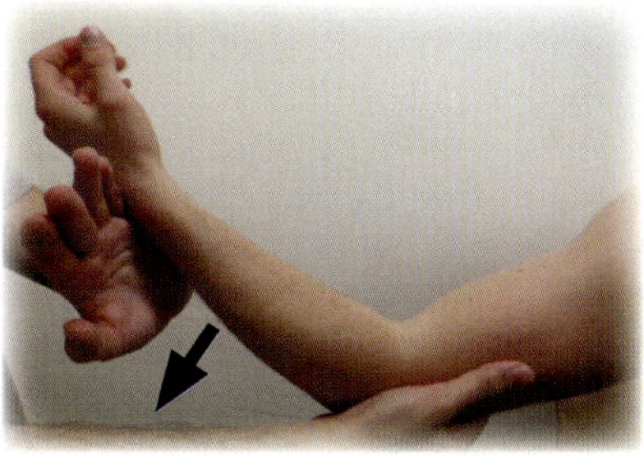

Fig 7.27 Testing the triceps brachii muscle through the extension of the forearm.

To test the function of the triceps brachii, ask the patient to extend their elbow whilst you resist the movement. You must also stabilise the elbow joint during this examination.
This is pictured in **Fig 7.27**.

To request this test from the patient ask them to: *"Straighten your elbow whilst I stabilise it and resist your movement by holding your forearm."*

6) Anterior muscles of the forearm

The anterior compartment of the forearm consists of eight muscles, which primarily focus on the flexion of the distal aspects of the upper limb. For ease of revision and understanding, we will divide the muscles into three groups based on their depth within the arm.

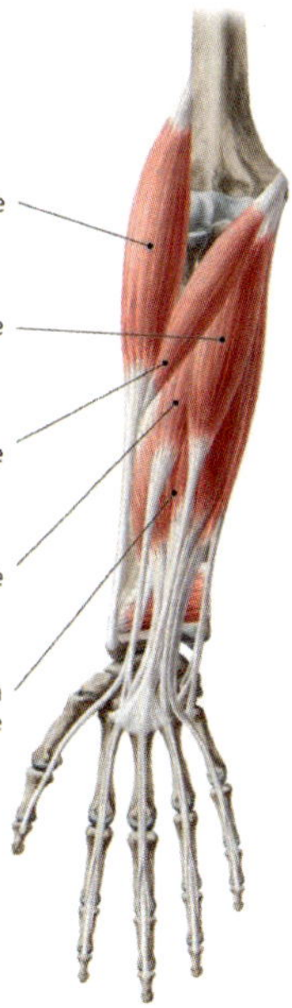

Fig 7.28 The superficial muscles of the anterior forearm.

The superficial muscles of the anterior compartment of the forearm are, from lateral to medial, the **pronator teres**, **flexor carpi radialis**, **palmaris longus**, and the **flexor carpi ulnaris**.

Pronator teres*

The pronator teres originates from both the humeral head and the ulnar head. Specifically, it originates from the medial epicondyle of the humerus (like all the other superficial flexors of the forearm) and coronoid process of the ulna, where it traverses under the brachioradialis (part of the posterior compartment of the arm) to attach to the pronator tuberosity on the lateral aspect of the shaft of the radius. Alongside the deeper pronator quadratus, it functions to **pronate the radius** about the ulna.
Similar to the other superficial flexors of the forearm, other than flexor carpi ulnaris, the pronator teres is innervated by the **median nerve**.[33]
Testing of this muscle is described and pictured with the pronator quadratus, in **Fig 7.35**.

Flexor carpi radialis*

More medially, the flexor carpi radialis (FCR) also originates from the common flexor tendon at the medial epicondyle of the humerus. **This is the point of origin for all the superficial and intermediate flexors of the forearm**.

The FCR then inserts at the base of the second and third metacarpal (of the index and middle finger) where it assists in the flexion and radial deviation (abduction) of the wrist. The muscle is appropriately named to help you remember information about it.

Palmaris longus*

The palmaris longus is the next medial superficial flexor of the forearm. It attaches to the **flexor retinaculum** (as described in carpal tunnel syndrome) and the **palmar aponeurosis** to weakly assist in the **flexion of the wrist joint**. Also **median nerve** innervated, this muscle is variable and is absent in many people.[63]

Flexor carpi ulnaris*

Finally, the flexor carpi ulnaris (FCU) arises from the **common flexor tendon** and attaches to the sesamoid carpal bone known as the **pisiform** (which sits inside the FCU tendon), the **hamate** carpal bone, and the **base of the fifth metacarpal** (of the little finger) The FCU assists in the **flexion and ulnar deviation** of the wrist.

The FCU is the only superficial muscle that is not innervated by the median nerve and is instead innervated by the ulnar nerve.[33,61]

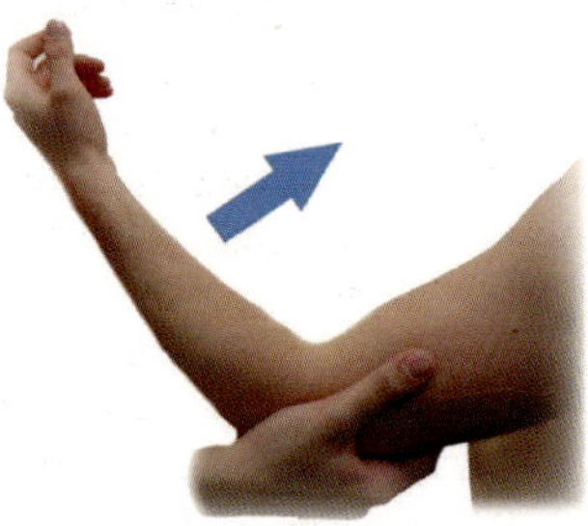

Fig 7.29 Flexion of the forearm.

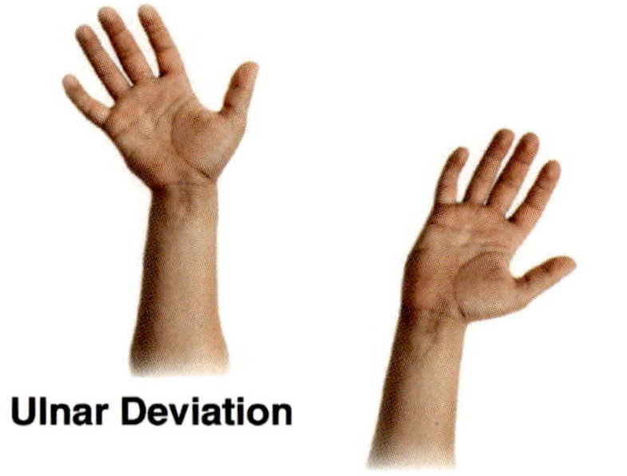

Fig 7.30 Radial and ulnar deviation of the wrist joint.

To generally test the superficial flexors of the anterior forearm, ask the patient to flex their elbows and hold it up like a boxer. Then, ask them to pronate their forearms to engage the pronator teres muscle. Finally, ask them to flex their wrists against resistance, which if successful, would lead to the patient's palms facing the floor. You, as the examiner, must provide resistance to the motion and stabilise the wrist joint.

The patient's motion is pictured in **Fig 7.31**.

To request this test from the patient ask them to: *"Can you make your arms like a boxer and bend your elbows in front of you. Then can you turn your wrists around and push down against my hands?"*

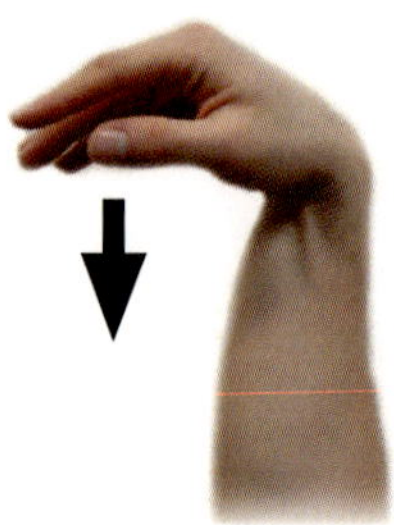

Fig 7.31 Testing of the superficial muscles of the anterior forearm through flexion of the wrist joint. This must be done against resistance provided by your hand and wrist joint stabilisation by grasping the forearm with your other hand.

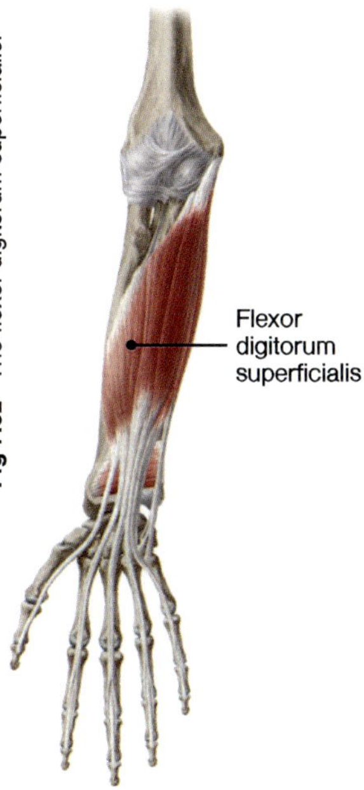

Fig 7.32 The flexor digitorum superficialis.

Flexor digitorum superficialis*

The intermediate layer of muscle within the anterior forearm consists only of the flexor digitorum superficialis (FDS). The FDS has two heads which originate from the common flexor tendon and the radius. It is between these two heads that the median nerve and ulnar artery passes through.[33,61] The FDS then travels distally where it gives off four tendons at the wrist, which travel through the carpal tunnel in a common flexor sheath (alongside the tendons of the flexor digitorum profundus) to attach to the four intermediate phalanges of the hand. It then assists in the **flexion of the wrist** and **flexes the metacarpophalangeal joints** and **proximal interphalangeal joints** of the last four digits. It is also innervated by the **median nerve**.[61,62]

To test the flexor digitorum superficialis, ask the patient to **flex their last four digits at the proximal interphalangeal joints** one at a time whilst you, as the examiner, provide resistance and stabilise the joint by grasping the proximal phalanx of the digit of you are testing at the time. Ideally, each digit would be tested individually whilst the other digits are stabilised, but this is much easier said than done. Alongside this, time constraints in the OSPE do not allow you to perform the most ideal test, and so it is accepted if you were to test all the tendons of the FDS at once by stabilising the medial four proximal interphalangeal joints and providing resistance to all four digits at once. This is the function test for the FDS that is advisable in the OSPE.

To request this test from the patient ask them:
"Can you bend the ends of your fingers whilst I provide resistance and hold the bottom parts?"

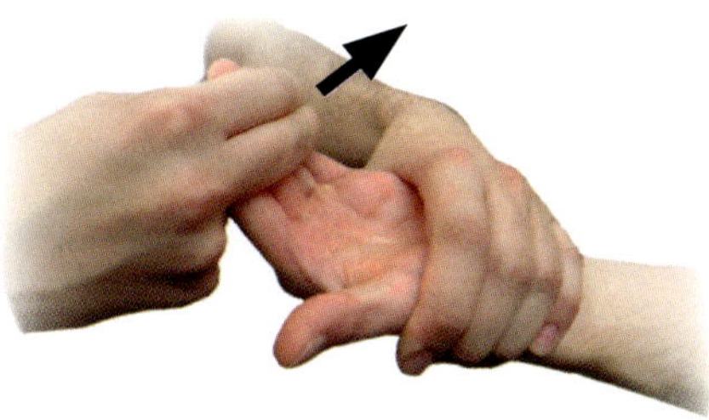

Fig 7.33 Testing of the flexor digitorum superficialis that should be conducted in the OSPE.

You are also able to test the function of the FDS, albeit not as accurately, by asking the patient to flex their medial four metacarpophalangeal joints against resistance. This is pictured in **Fig 7.33**, but is the not the go-test for the FDS as it also tests other muscles.

To request this test from the patient ask them to:
"Can you bend your fingers whilst I provide resistance and hold the front bit of your hand?"

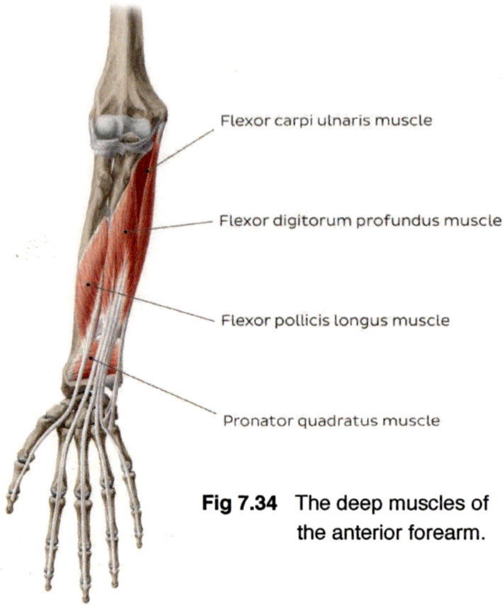

Fig 7.34 The deep muscles of the anterior forearm.

The deep muscles of the anterior aspect of the forearm consist of the final three muscles we will discuss in this section: The **flexor pollicis longus**, **flexor digitorum profundus**, and the **pronator quadratus**.

Flexor pollicis longus

The flexor pollicis longus (FPL) lies laterally to the flexor digitorum profundus (FDP) and it originates from the shaft of the radius and surrounding interosseous membrane (pictured in **Fig 7.34**). It then attaches to the base of the distal phalanx of the first digit (thumb) and works in the flexion of its interphalangeal joint through it's tendon which travels through the carpal tunnel alongside the tendons of FDS and FDP. Remember that the thumb only has one interphalangeal joint, as opposed to the other four digits which have two. FPL is also innervated by the median nerve.[61,62]

Flexor digitorum profundus*

The FDP originates from the ulna and associated interosseous membrane. At the wrist, it splits into four tendons that pass through the carpal tunnel in the common flexor sheath (alongside the tendons of the FDS and FPL) and attach to the distal phalanges of the last four digits. It functions in the **flexion of the distal interphalangeal joint** of these fingers, and assists in the **flexion of the metacarpophalangeal joints** and the wrist, much like FDS. Furthermore, it lies deep to the FDS but traverses more distally through the splittings at the end of the tendons of the FDS, known as Camper's Chiasms. The FDP is innervated by the **ulnar nerve (the medial two tendons)** and the **median nerve (the lateral two tendons)**.[61,62]

To test the FDP, ask the patient to flex their last four digits at the distal interphalangeal joints against resistance. Ideally, each finger should be done individually, and you, as the examiner, should stabilise the distal interphalangeal joints and provide resistance to their motion.

Pronator quadratus*

Finally, the pronator quadratus originates from the distal aspect of the ulnar shaft and inserts into the adjacent area of the radial shaft. It is involved in the **pronation of the radius**, alongside pronator teres, and is innervated by the **median nerve**.[33,62]

To test the pronator quadratus (and the pronator teres), ask the patient to pronate their forearm against resistance, whilst you, as the examiner, stabilise the wrist joint by holding the patients elbow or forearm.

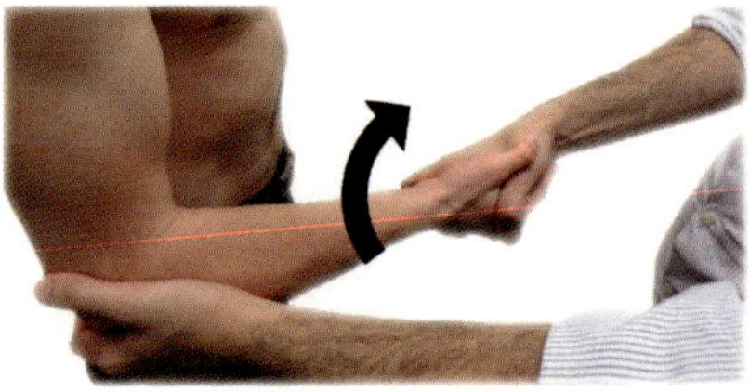

Fig 7.35 Testing the pronator teres and the pronator quadratus through the pronation of the forearm.

7) Posterior muscles of the forearm

There are eleven muscles of the posterior compartment of the forearm which are primarily extensors of the wrist joint and joints of the hand. They are all innervated by the **radial nerve** and can be grouped based on depth within the forearm. We will briefly discuss some of these muscles, but none are needed to be known in as significant a detail as in the anterior compartment of the forearm.

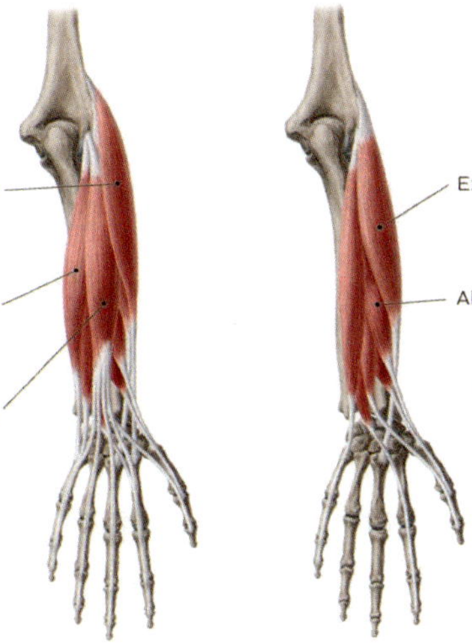

Fig 7.36 The superficial muscles of the posterior forearm.

The superficial muscles of the posterior compartment of the forearm, beginning laterally, are the **brachioradialis**, **extensor carpi radialis longus**, **extensor carpi radialis brevis**, **extensor digitorum**, **extensor digiti minimi**, **extensor carpi ulnaris**, and the **anconeus**.

Pictured in **Fig 7.36**, the **brachioradialis** is a superficial muscle that is an anomaly in the posterior compartment of the forearm in that it works at **flexion of the elbow joint**. Depending on the position of the forearm, it is also capable of pronation and supination.

The **anconeus** is a small triangle shaped muscle that originates from the lateral epicondyle of the humerus and inserts into the olecranon and posterior surface of the ulna. It weakly agonises the actions of the triceps brachii in that it weakly assists in the extension of the elbow joint, and like all the muscles of the posterior compartment of the forearm, it is innervated by the **radial nerve**.[33,62]

There are five muscles in the deep compartment of the posterior forearm.
From lateral to medial, **the supinator**, **abductor pollicis longus**, **extensor pollicis brevis**, **extensor pollicis longus**, and the **extensor indicis**. Again, knowing that they are all innervated by the radial nerve is enough, as you are easily able to work out the functions of the muscles through their names.

Appropriately named, the supinator supinates the forearm.

In fact, it is useful to know that pollicis = thumb, indicis = index finger, digiti minimi = little finger, brevis = short, longus = long, and digitorum = fingers. This will help you work out the function of certain muscles and their attachments.

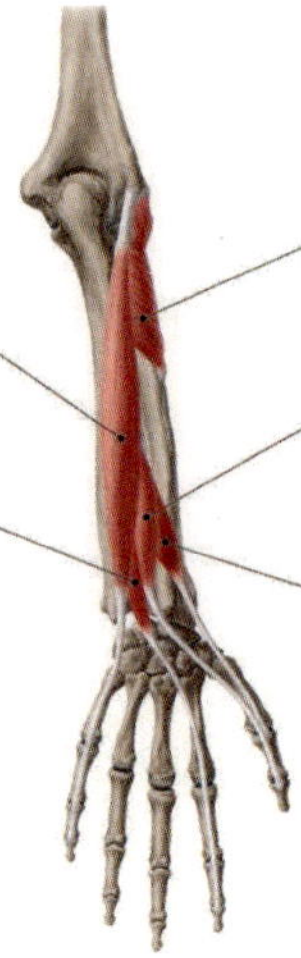

Fig 7.37 The deep muscles of the posterior forearm.

Two tests exist for the assessment of the function of the muscles in the posterior compartment of the forearm.

The first test assesses the function of the extensors of the wrist by asking the patient to **flatten their hand** and **extend their wrist's back against resistance.** You, as the examiner, should stabilise the wrist joint and provide appropriate resistance. This is pictured in **Fig 7.38**.

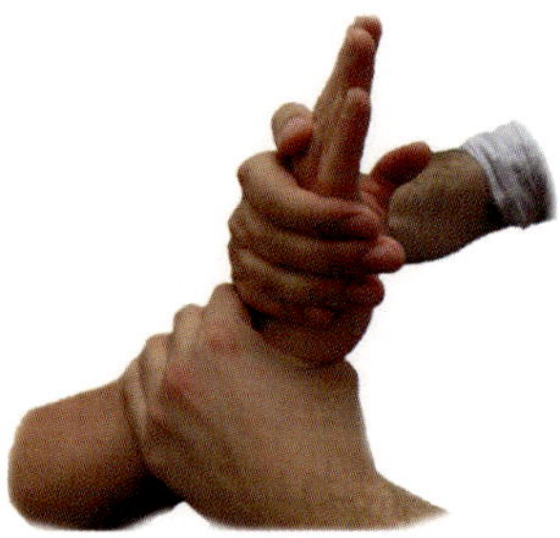

Fig 7.38 Testing of the wrist extensor muscles in the posterior compartment of the forearm.

The second test involves asking the patient to extend their fingers whilst they hand is positioned on a flat surface to assess the function of the extensors of the digits.

To request this test from the patient ask them to:

"Can you straighten your hand and try to bend your wrist back whilst I resist you?"

or

"Can you place your hands flat on the table/bed for me, and then raise your fingers up?"

8) Intrinsic muscles of the hand

The intrinsic muscles of the hand consist of the **interossei**, lumbricals, **thenar muscles**, **hypothenar muscles**, and the adductor pollicis.[65]

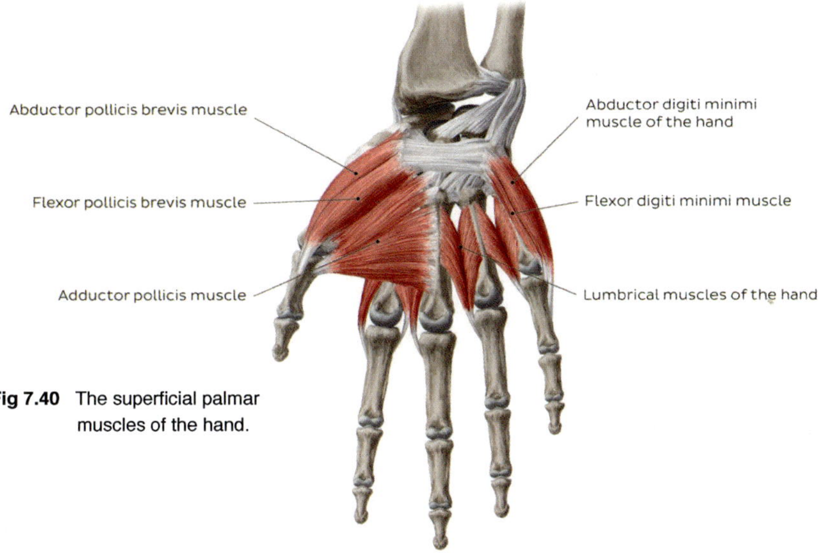

Fig 7.40 The superficial palmar muscles of the hand.

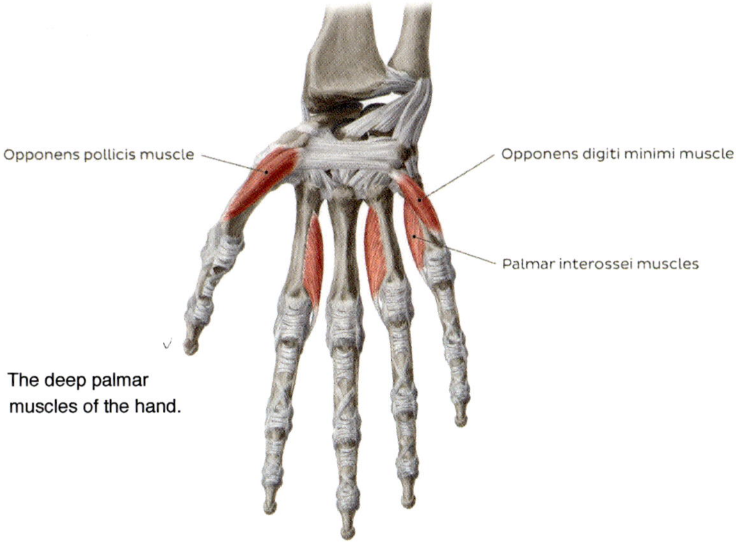

Fig 7.41 The deep palmar muscles of the hand.

Interossei muscles*

The interossei muscles are located **between the metacarpal bones** of the hand and are grouped based on the surface of their location. They are all innervated by the **ulnar nerve**, and they all originate from the metacarpals and insert into the respective proximal phalanges of the digit upon which they function.

The three **palmar interossei** are located deep on the palmar side of the hand, and they function to **adduct the digits** at the metacarpophalangeal joints due to their origins on the metacarpals being proximally located to the midline of the hand (the midline of the third digit).

The four **dorsal interossei** are located superficially on the dorsal surface of the hand and work to **abduct the digits** at the metacarpophalangeal joints. This is because they are attached on the distal end of the metacarpals relative to the midline of the hand (though they vary in the radial side and ulnar side attachment, much like the palmar interossei).

To test the palmar interossei, place a piece of paper between each of the four medial digits of the patients hand, and ask them to adduct their digits as hard as they can to stop you, as the examiner, from pulling the piece of paper from between their fingers. This is pictured in **Fig 7.42**.

Believe it or not, this is a test that can be asked about in the OSPE.

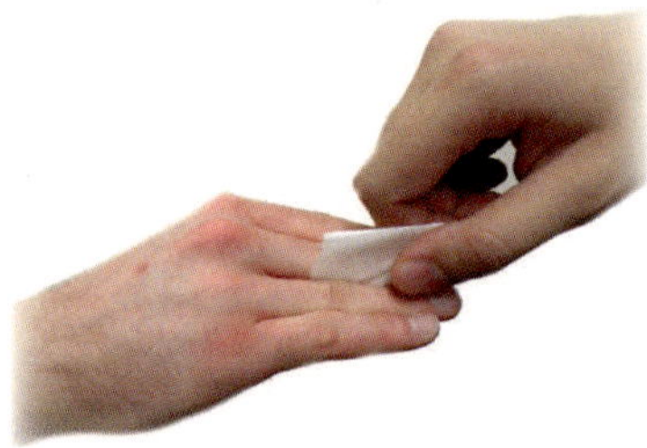

Fig 7.42 The test for the palmar interrossei.

To test the dorsal interossei, ask the patient to adduct each of the four medial digits one by one, whilst you, as the examiner, provide resistance and stabilise the metacarpophalangeal joints by holding the proximal end of the patients hand. This is pictured in **7.43**, and this is a test that is more likely to be asked of you than the test for the palmar interossei.

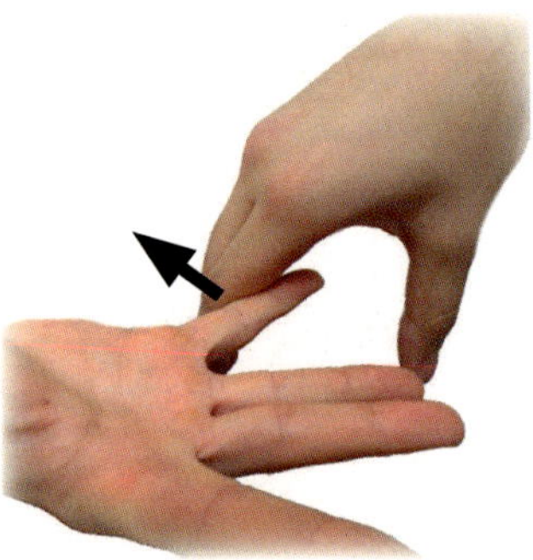

Fig 7.43 The test for the dorsal interrossei.

Lumbricals

The four lumbricals of the hand originate from the radial side of the respective FDP tendons (although the bipennate lumbricals of the third and fourth digits also have a head originating from the ulnar side of the tendon). They work to flex the metacarpophalangeal joints and extend the interphalangeal joints in the hand. The lumbricals of the second and third digits are innervated by the median nerve, and the lumbricals of the fourth and fifth digits are innervated by the ulnar nerve.[65]

Paralysis of the medial two lumbricals as a result of ulnar neuropathy can, therefore, lead to a deformity known as the ulnar claw, where there is a hyperextension of the metacarpophalangeal joints and flexion at the interphalangeal joints of the 4th and 5th digits.[66]

Thenar muscles*

The thenar muscles are three muscles located at the base of the thumb which produce a bulge, known as the thenar eminence. They are responsible for the fine movements of the thumb and are innervated by the median nerve.[33,65]
These muscles are the flexor pollicis brevis, the abductor pollicis brevis, and the opponens pollicis.

Hypothenar muscles*

The hypothenar muscles are the abductor digiti minimi, the flexor digiti minimi brevis, and the opponens digiti minimi, and all function for the fine control of the fifth digit (the little finger). They are innervated by the ulnar nerve and produce a bulge proximally and medially under the fifth digit, known as the hypothenar eminence.

Both the thenar and the hypothenar muscles can be tested together, by asking the patient to touch their thumb to their little finger as hard as they can. This is pictured in **Fig 7.44**. You, as the examiner, should then try to disconnect the thumb and the little finger by trying to pass your thumb (in an upwards motion) through the point of connection between the two fingers. This is a likely test that you can be asked to perform in the OSPE.

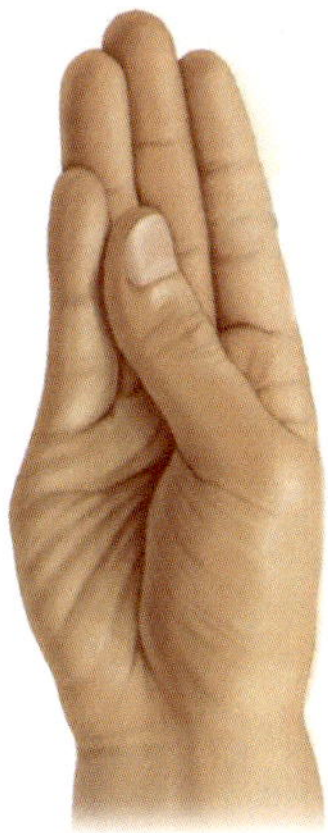

Fig 7.44 The positioning of the patient's fingers when testing the thenar and hypothenar muscles.

Adductor pollicis

The adductor pollicis is innervated by the ulnar nerve, and, appropriately named, it adducts the thumb.[33,65]

9) Sternocleidomastoid

Finally, it is appropriate to the discuss the sternocleidomastoid (SCM) muscle at the end of this learning objective. This is because the SCM is not linked to the upper limb other than the fact it attaches to the clavicle, but it is a muscle that can appropriately be asked about in the upper limb station of the OSPE.

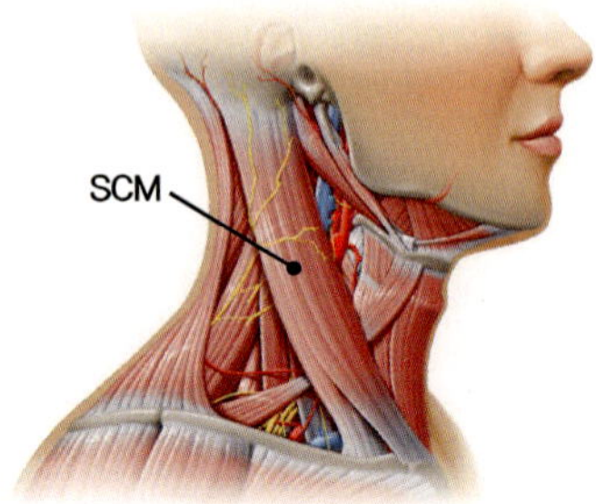

Fig 7.45 The sternocleidomastoid muscle in situ.

The sternocleidomastoid, appropriately named, originates from the **sternal manubrium** and the **medial third of the clavicle**, and it attaches to the **mastoid process** of the temporal bone. It functions to **rotate the head** to the opposite side when unilaterally contracting. However, contraction of both SCMs will result in the **flexion of the neck** and **extension of the head** at the atlanto-occipital joint (bending the neck forwards whilst tilting the head back).

Much like the trapezius, the SCM is also innervated by **CN XI, the accessory nerve**, and testing of this muscle is conducted during the testing of the cranial nerves.[67]

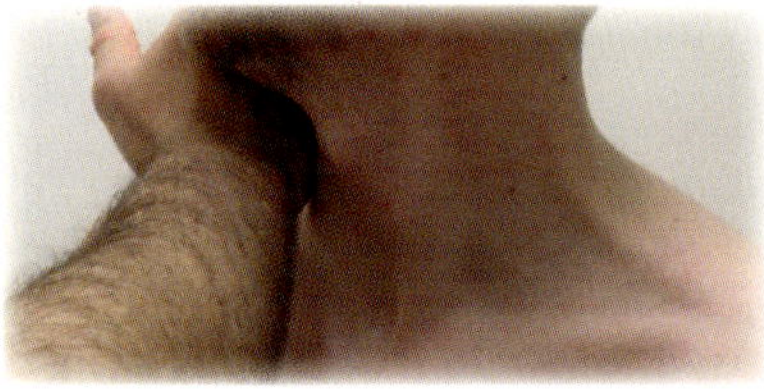

Fig 7.46 Testing of the SCM by resisting rotation of the patients head.

As a result, Samuel Hammond has discussed the testing of the SCM in the chapter previous to this. However, for the sake of continuity of knowledge for the upper limb station, the SCM is tested by placing the dorsal aspect of your hand laterally on the patient's cheek, and asking the patient to turn their head to the side of your hand, resisting the pressure you are exerting in the direction opposite to their movement. At the same time, palpate the ipsilateral sternocleidomastoid with your other hand. Repeat this procedure with the contralateral SCM.

Extra medical notes

Although it is a rarity for students to be asked about the graded strength of a muscle in the OSPE assessments, it is good practice to begin assessing this from early on. This is because it is extremely useful when conducting limb neurological examinations in your clinical placements and future practice. The following scale by the Medical Research Counci, is used to grade the strength of a muscle:[68]

- 0: No clinically observable muscle contraction
- 1: No movement but a slight visible or palpable contraction of the muscle
- 2: Limb movement, but not against gravity
- 3: Movement against gravity but not resistance
- 4: Movement against at least some resistance supplied by the examiner
- 5: Full strength

The difficulty with this and similar scales is the large range in strength possible between grades 4 and 5.

3 The nerve supply to the upper limb

Brachial plexus

The brachial plexus is the network that innervates the skin and musculature of the upper limb. It is formed in the root of the neck, and it is theoretically divided into five parts as it transcends into the upper limb. At the level of the OSPEs, this is purely to aid the understanding of the development of the five main terminal nerve branches of the upper limb.

The five parts that the brachial plexus is divided into are, from proximal to distal; **roots**, **trunks**, **divisions**, **cords**, and **branches**.
A mnemonic for this is '**Roman Traitors Daggered Caesar's Back**'.

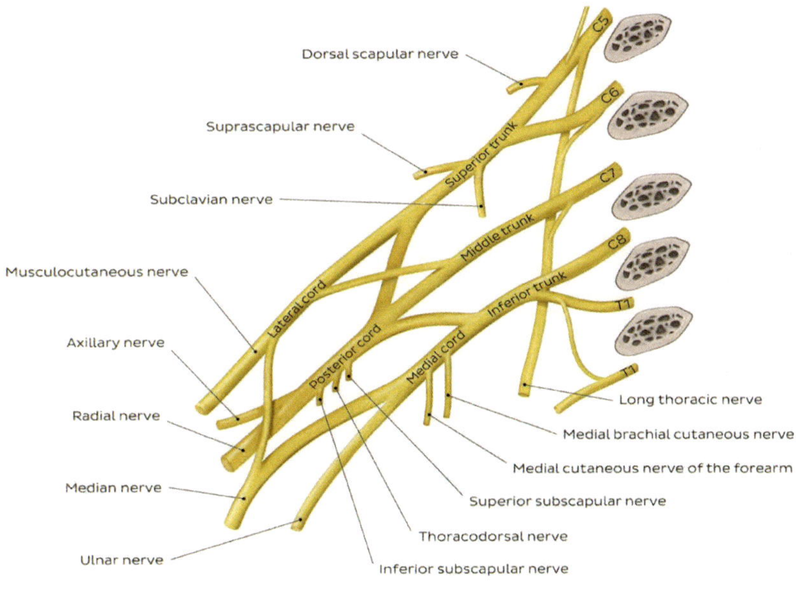

Fig 7.47 Summary of the structure and branches of the brachial plexus.

Spinal nerve roots

The brachial plexus is formed by the anterior rami of the four lower cervical and the first thoracic nerve roots (**C5, C6, C7, C8, T1**). This is what is meant by roots.

These five spinal nerves then converge together to form **three trunks**.
C5 and C6 spinal nerves converge to form the superior trunk, C8 and T1 converge to form the inferior trunk, and C7 becomes the middle trunk.[33]

Further lateral, the three trunks each divide into two divisions, the **anterior and the posterior divisions**, depending on the direction of the nerves. These **six divisions** continue into the axilla and combine to form **cords**.

The posterior cord is formed from the combination of the posterior divisions of the superior, middle, and inferior trunks.
The anterior divisions of the superior and middle trunks combine to form the lateral cord. The anterior division of the inferior trunk continues and forms the medial cord.

The cords can then divide and combine to form the five major **branches** that continue down as the nerve supply for all the motor function and sensation of the upper limb.

The **musculocutaneous nerve (spinal roots C5, C6, and C7)** arises from the lateral cord and it innervates the **coracobrachialis**, the **brachialis**, and the **biceps brachii** muscle before continuing on to become the lateral cutaneous nerve of the forearm.
Motor testing, therefore, involves **flexion of the forearm** against resistance.

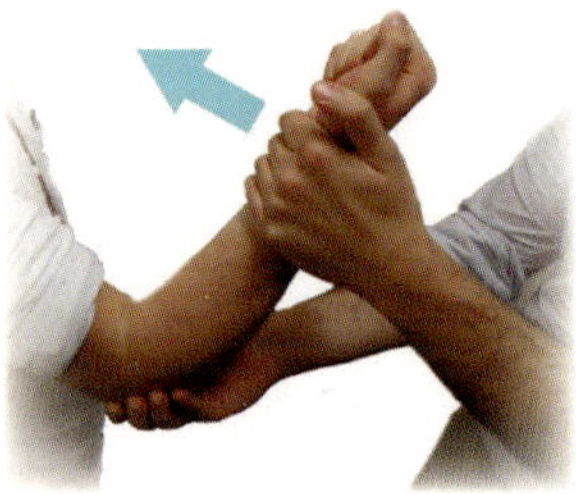

Fig 7.48 Motor testing of the musculocutaneous nerve through flexion of the forearm against resistance.

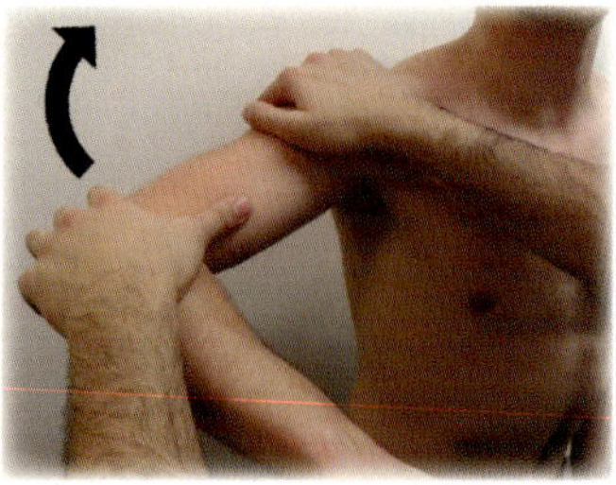

Fig 7.49 Motor testing of the axillary nerve through abduction of the arms against resistance.

The **axillary nerve (C5 and C6)** is one of the branches to arise from the division of the posterior cord, and it innervates the **teres minor** and **deltoid muscles**.
Motor testing, therefore, involves asking the patient to **abduct their arms against resistance**.

The **median nerve (C6, C7, C8, and T1)** arises from the combination of the lateral and medial cords, and it innervates the **flexor muscles in the forearm** (apart from the flexor carpi ulnaris and the medial aspect of the flexor digitorum profundus), **the thenar muscles**, and the **two lateral lumbricals** associated with the second and third digits.

Testing of the median nerve's motor function, therefore, involves **wrist flexion, wrist abduction, and flexion of fingers** at the proximal interphalangeal joints against resistance. It also involves thenar muscle flexion and abduction.

The **radial nerve** arises from the posterior cord and **all the spinal roots (C5-T1)** and travels posteriorly in the upper limb to innervate the **posterior compartments of the arm** and forearm in a cutaneous and motor manner. It continues down to provide skin innervation to the **posterolateral aspect of the hand.** Motor testing, therefore, involves **extension at the elbow joint, wrist joint, and metacarpophalangeal joints** against resistance.

The **ulnar nerve (C8 and T1)** is the other branch that arises from the division of the posterior cord and it innervates the **flexor carpi ulnaris, the medial half of flexor digitorum profundus, and the muscles of the hand** (apart from the thenar muscles and two lateral lumbricals).

Motor function testing, therefore, involves **abduction and adduction of digits,** and **flexion and ulnar deviation at the wrist joint** against resistance.

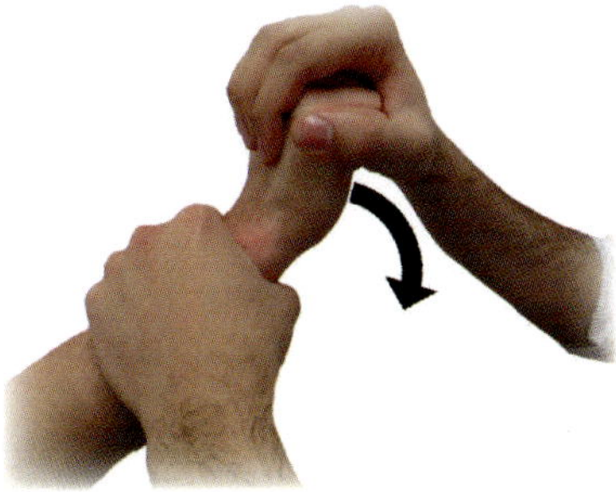

Fig 7.50 Motor testing of the median nerve through wrist flexion.

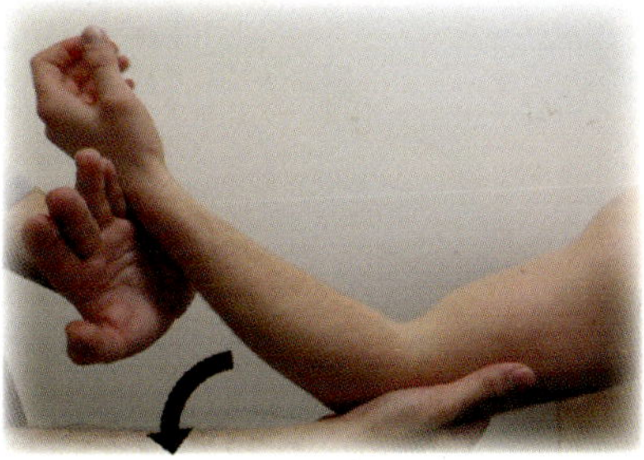

Fig 7.51 Motor testing of the radial nerve through elbow extension.

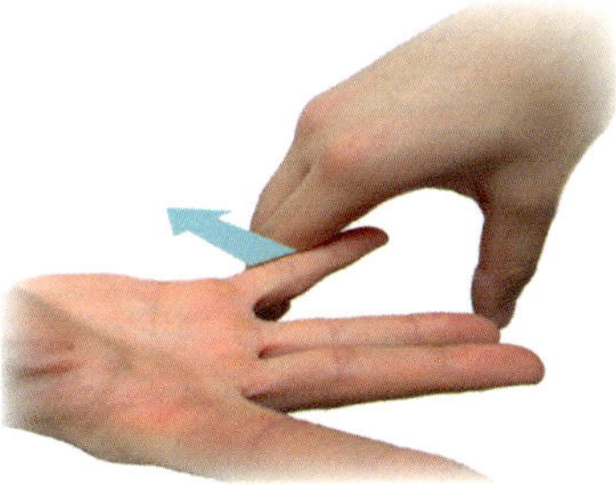

Fig 7.52 Motor testing of the ulnar nerve through abduction of the digits.

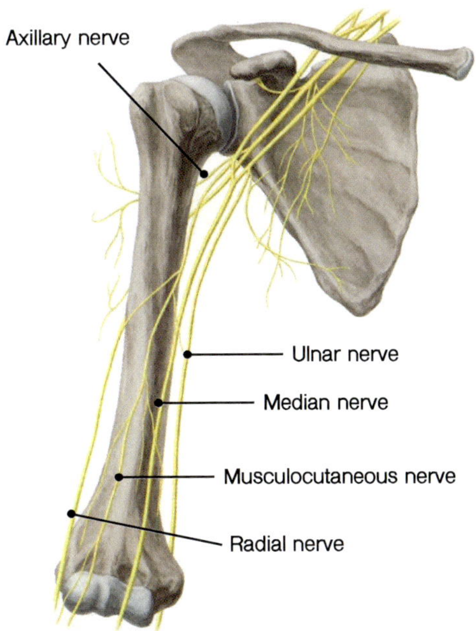

Fig 7.53 The nerves of the upper arm.

Extra medical notes

Two notable brachial plexus pathologies for pre-clinical education are **Erb-Duchenne palsy** and **Dejerine–Klumpke palsy**.[69]

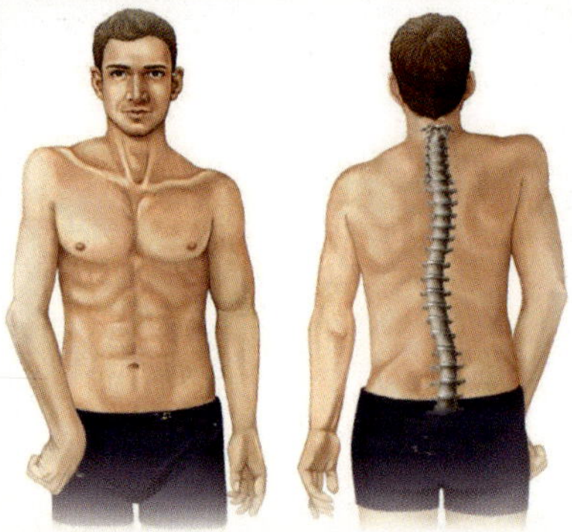

Erb's palsy results from upper brachial plexus injury involving spinal nerve roots C5 and C6, and therefore the suprascapular, axillary, and musculocutaneous nerve.[70] This results in a typical Erb's palsy patient presenting with loss of lateral sensation in the arm and paralysis of the deltoid, biceps, coracobrachialis and brachialis muscles.[33] Erb's Palsy can result from an increase in the angle between the shoulder and head, which can excessively stretch the nerve roots of C5 and C6.

Fig 7.54 Illustration of a patient presenting with Erb's palsy.

Klumpke's palsy results from lower brachial plexus injury involving spinal nerve roots C8 and T1, which stems from hyperabduction of the arm.[33] This, therefore, effects the ulnar and median nerves, and patients present with loss of medial sensation in the arm and loss of motor function in the intrinsic hand muscles, FCU, and FDP.[71] Classically, the most notable symptom is the claw-hand, caused by hyperextension of the metacarpophalangeal joints and flexion at the interphalangeal joints of the 4th and 5th digits.[65]

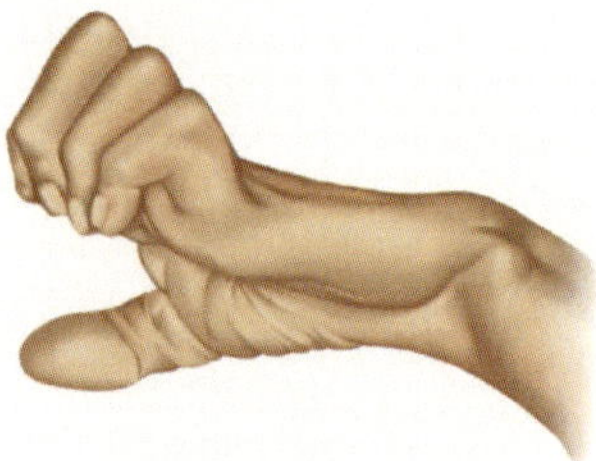

Fig 7.55 Hyperextension of the metacarpophalangeal joints and flexion at the interphalangeal joints - claw hand.

Sensory testing of peripheral nerves

It is vital to recognise the difference between dermatomes and cutaneous innervation.

A dermatome is the area of skin supplied by a single dorsal root of the spinal cord. This area, however, may be supplied by a number of different nerves that either wholly or partly originate from that particular part of the spinal cord.

In contrast, cutaneous innervation is an area of skin that is specifically innervated by that nerve, which may originate from numerous dorsal roots of the spinal cord.

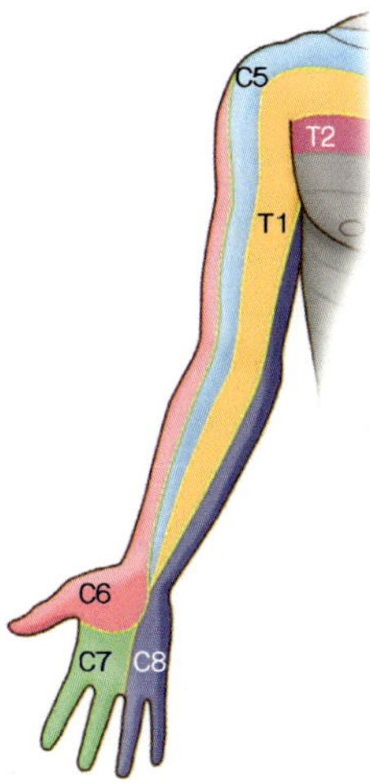

Fig 7.56 Dermatomes of the upper limb

In a clinical setting, one assesses the neurological integrity of skin sensation using light touch, pin-prick, proprioception, and vibration.

However, within the OSPE, simple **light-touch sensation** (and perhaps pin-prick sensation at a push) are expected to be the only modalities tested.

Light-touch sensation

Using the wisp of the cotton wool, touch the patient's sternum to establish a central baseline sensation and ask them to confirm once they can feel it.

Then ask the patient close their eyes and to say 'yes' once they feel the wisp of cotton wool touch the skin on their upper limb. It is recommended to begin testing from the C5 dermatome, and to work around the upper limb until the T2 dermatome.

Also assess the contralateral dermatome on the other side of the body before continuing on that limb, and ask the patient whether the sensation felt was the same on both sides.

The comparison of corresponding dermatomes and peripheral nerves on both sides is essential in upper limb sensation testing.

Pin-prick sensation testing, which assesses the spinothalamic tracts, is conducted using the same method as described for light touch sensation, only a neurotip is used in the place of cotton wool.

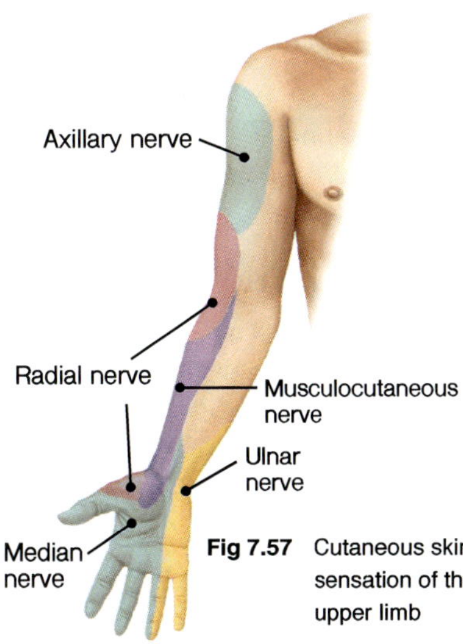

Fig 7.57 Cutaneous skin sensation of the upper limb

However, for the individual testing of the cutaneous nerves, please refer to **Fig 7.57** for guidance on anatomical locations.

Reflexes

The two reflexes of interest in the upper limb OSPE are the biceps brachii tendon and the triceps brachii tendon reflex, both of which are stretch reflexes.

The stretch reflex is the rapid physiological response by a muscle designed as a protective measure against over-stretch. To prevent tearing, the muscle (and the agonistic group of muscles) contracts as a result of an impulse that is sent along the reflex arc, which is not cortically controlled, to the spinal cord and back. This also leads to an inhibition of the antagonistic muscles, which leads to their relaxation.

Biceps tendon reflex

This is performed by striking the biceps brachii tendon within the cubital fossa, which should lead to elbow flexion.

As the examiner, place your thumb on the tendon of the partially contracted biceps brachii in the cubital fossa of a partially flexed elbow.
You must also support the patient's arm, and this technique is pictured in **Fig 7.58**.

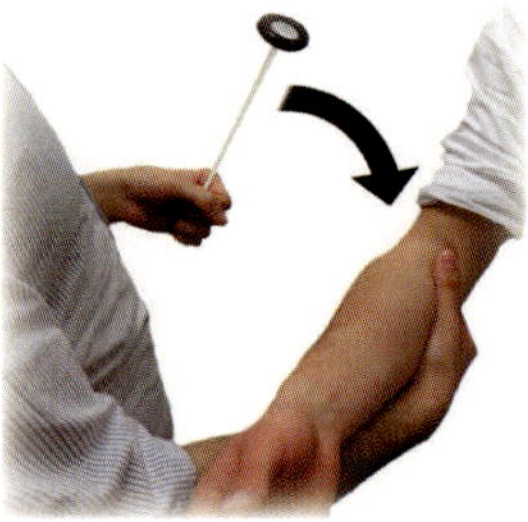

Fig 7.58 Eliciting the biceps brachii tendon reflex.

Then, with a brisk motion, strike your thumb with the tendon hammer to elicit a response from the biceps brachii and its synergistic muscles.

This test assesses the function of the **musculocutaneous nerve**, and so **spinal nerve roots C5 and C6**. If intact, a brief and rapid contraction of the biceps brachii will be observed. An absent or weaker than appropriate response/ contraction, known as a diminished reflex, is indicative of a lower motor neurone lesion.[72]

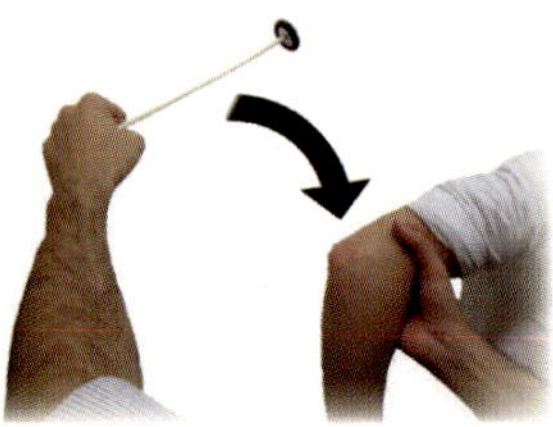

Fig 7.59 Eliciting the triceps brachii tendon reflex.

Triceps tendon reflex

This is performed by striking the triceps brachii tendon located just superiorly to the olecranon process of the elbow, which should lead to elbow extension.

As the examiner, support the patients partially flexed arm and elbow as pictured in **Fig 7.59**.
Then, with a brisk motion of the tendon hammer, strike the triceps tendon to elicit a response from the triceps brachii. This also inhibits the flexor muscles of the forearm.
This test assesses the function of the radial nerve, and so spinal nerve roots C7 and C8. If intact, a brief and rapid contraction of the triceps brachii will be observed.

Extra medical notes

As mentioned, brisk reflexes are indicative of an upper motor neurone lesion.[72] The two notable pathologies where this is observed are multiple sclerosis and stroke.[73] Multiple sclerosis is a disease where there is degeneration of the myelin within the CNS, and stroke results from a disruption in blood flow to regions of the brain.

Degeneration of motor and sensory neurones in Charcot Marie Tooth disease is an example of lower motor neurone disease which leads to weak and diminished reflexes.

4 The arterial supply to the upper limb

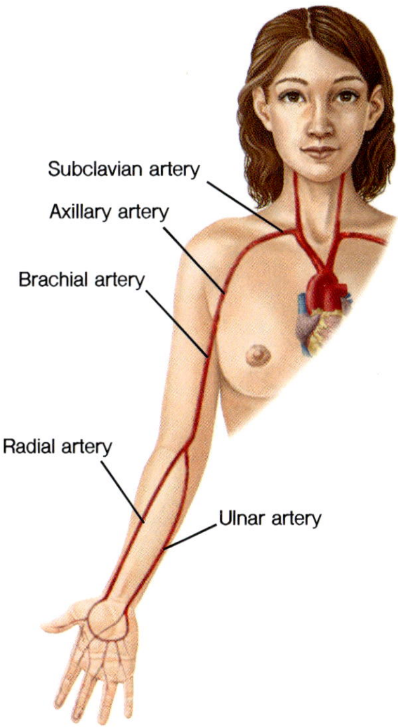

Fig 7.60 The key arteries of in the upper limb.

The blood supply to the upper limb begins with the **subclavian artery**. The right subclavian artery arises from the brachiocephalic trunk and the left subclavian artery is the third branch of the aortic arch.
The subclavian then travels between the anterior and middle scalene muscles, and as it crosses the lateral border of the first rib, it becomes the **axillary artery**.

The subclavian pulse can be palpated anywhere superiorly and just posterior to the proximal tip and midline of the clavicle as it can be **compressed against rib I**.

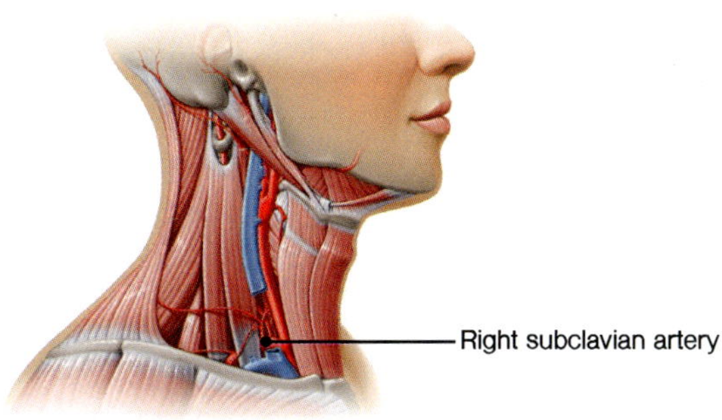

Fig 7.61 The subclavian artery.

The **axillary artery** is a large vessel that lies deep to the pectoralis minor and travels down the axilla to the **inferior border of the teres major** where it becomes the **brachial artery**. It is protected in the axillary fascia, which is a neurovascular bundle comprising of the axillary artery and the cords of the brachial plexus, and the suspensory ligaments which attach to the fascia. Out of the several branches that arise from the axillary artery, of note in the OSPE are the anterior and posterior humeral circumflex arteries which wrap around the surgical neck of the humerus and are frequently damaged in cases of humeral fracture.[33]
This may be a potential recall question.

The pulsation of the artery can be felt by deep palpation of the axilla after abducting the arm. However, for the purposes of the OSPE, it is unexpected for you to be asked to demonstrate palpation of the subclavian or axillary artery.

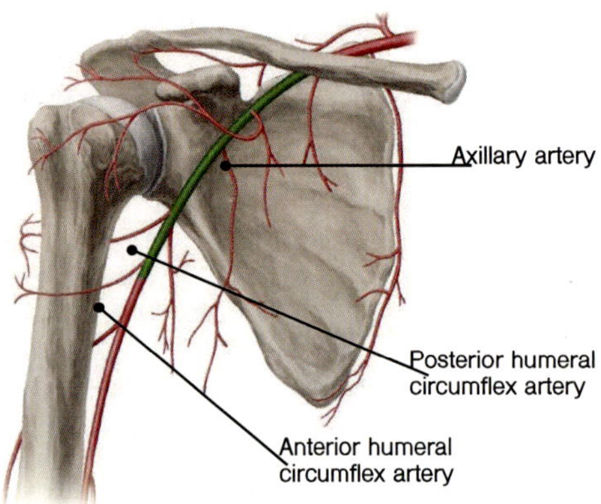

Fig 7.62 The axillary artery highlighted in green for ease of viewing.

The **brachial artery** stems from the axillary artery at the inferior border of teres major and continues down as the main supply of blood for the arm.

Just distal to the axillary artery, the brachial artery gives rise to the profunda brachii artery branch, which travels deep and supplies the posterior compartment of the arm.

The brachial artery travels anteriorly down the arm and supplies the **biceps brachii, coracobrachialis, and the brachialis** before reaching the cubital fossa where it bifurcates into the **radial and ulnar arteries**.

Its pulse can be palpated in the mid-arm and the cubital fossa, as described by *Arian Arjomandi Rad* in the *CVS chapter*.

However, for continuity of knowledge for the upper limb station, the brachial artery pulsation in the mid-arm can be palpated on the medial side of the arm between the biceps brachii and the triceps brachii tendon, and the cubital fossa pulsation can be palpated medially to the biceps brachii tendon. In both locations, the brachial artery is **compressed against the humerus**.

The ulnar artery is one of the two terminal branches that arise from the brachial artery, and it terminates at the anastomosis with the radial artery at the superficial palmar arch (supplied predominantly by the ulnar artery) and deep palmar arch (supplied predominantly by the radial artery). It also supplies the anteromedial aspect of the forearm and enters the hand anteriorly to the flexor retinaculum. Its pulse can be located by pressing the ulnar artery on the **head of the ulna.**

The **radial artery** is the second terminal branch originating from the brachial artery, supplying the posterolateral aspect of the forearm before travelling posteriorly through the anatomical snuffbox to give rise to rise to the deep palmar arch and branches which supply the thumb, index finger and the superficial palmar arch. Its pulse can be palpated by compressing the radial artery onto the **radial bone**, immediately lateral to the prominent tendon of the flexor carpi radialis.

As described by *Arian Arjomandi Rad*, you have to note the pulse rate and rhythm when asked to demonstrate palpation for a particular pulse in the OSPE. You simply have to note whether the pulse has a normal (sinus) rhythm or is irregular, and time the pulse has to be measured for is 15 seconds. You must then multiply this by four to give you the pulse in beats per minute.

The Allen test

In order to determine if it is safe to take blood, the patient is asked to perform an Allen test.[74] This involves asking the patient to clench their fist for 30 seconds whilst the health care professional applies occlusive pressure to the patient's two arteries simultaneously to block off the blood supply to the hand. Once the hand is opened, the time taken for the hand to flush back to the normal colour is measured to determine the **blood flow of the ulnar artery**.[74] You will not be required to physically do this test in the OSPE, but knowledge of this procedure is important.

5 The venous drainage of the upper limb

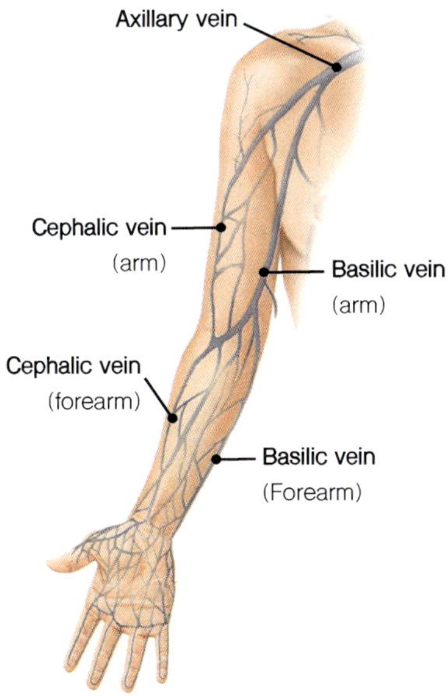

Fig 7.63 The veins of the upper limb

The venous drainage of the upper limb can be divided into the systems of the **superficial and deep veins**.

Both of these venous systems interconnect with one another throughout the upper limb through perforating veins, and we will discuss this in a fashion opposite to the arteries of the upper limb, as veins originate distally in the venous networks of the hand and return blood to the subclavian vein proximally.

The deep veins of the arm and forearm accompany the path of the arteries up until the axillary vein, where they join the superficial veins of the forearm and return all blood from the upper limb to the subclavian vein. The deep veins of the upper limb also form venae comitantes around the arteries of the upper limb and are, therefore, named after them. The most prominent of these deep veins are the brachial veins in the upper arm, which develop in pairs around each brachial artery.

The two prominent superficial veins of the upper limb are the **basilic** and **cephalic veins**, which both originate from the dorsal venous network of the hand.

The **cephalic vein** ascends from the anatomical snuffbox along the **radial side** of the upper limb, laterally to the biceps brachii. It then joins the axillary vein superior to the pectoralis minor muscle.

The **basilic vein** ascends up the **ulnar side** of the arm, medial to the biceps brachii, and joins the brachial veins to form the axillary veins.

The basilic and cephalic veins are connected by the median cubital vein at the elbow joint.

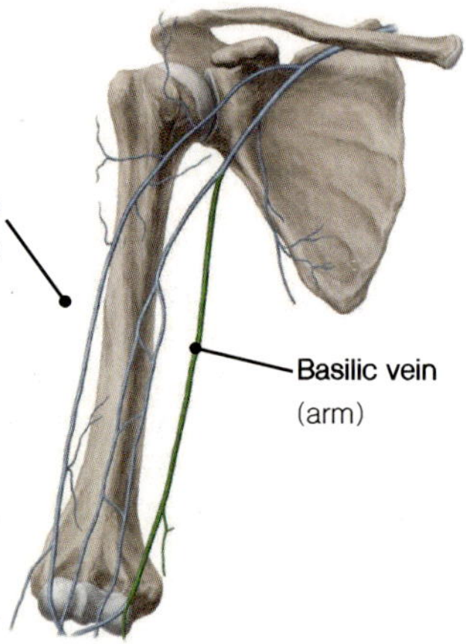

Fig 7.64 The veins of the arm
(basilic vein highlighted in green)

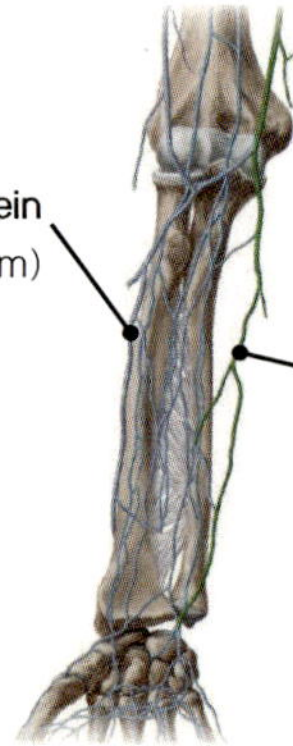

Fig 7.65 The veins of the forearm
(basilic vein highlighted in green)

6 Borders and contents of the relevant upper limb structures

For the OSPE, you are required to know the boundaries and contents of the axilla, the cubital fossa, the anatomical snuff-box, and the carpal tunnel.

The axilla

The axilla is the region between the upper limb and the thorax, inferior to the glenohumeral joint.
Its borders are created by the **pectoralis major** and **minor** anteriorly; the **thoracic wall** and the **serratus anterior** medially; the **subscapularis**, **latissimus dorsi**, and **teres major** posteriorly; and the **intertubercular sulcus** of the humerus laterally.

It contains the **axillary artery, axillary vein, brachial plexus, axillary lymph nodes, the tendon of the short head of the biceps brachii, and the tendon of the coracobrachialis.**

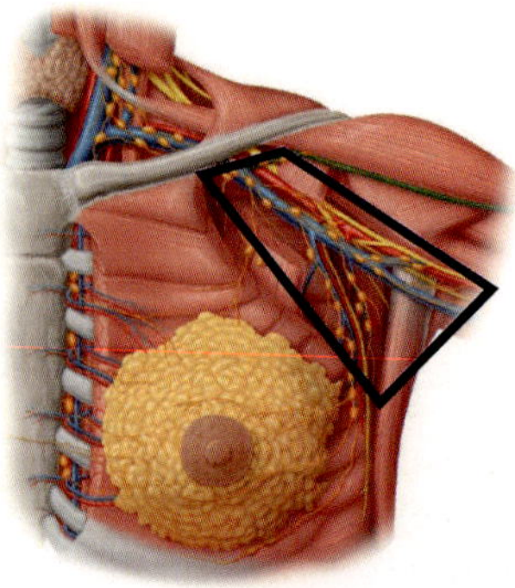

Fig 7.66 The axilla and it's contents.

The cubital fossa

The cubital fossa is a shallow wedge-shaped depression anterior to the elbow joint.

It's lateral border is formed by the **brachioradialis**; it's medial border is formed by the **pronator teres**; and it's superior border is formed by an imaginery line between the **epicondyles of the humerus**.
The floor of the cubital fossa is formed by the **brachialis**, and the roof is formed by the **bicipital aponeurosis**, fasica, and skin.

It contains, from lateral to medial: **the radial nerve, biceps tendon, brachial artery, and median nerve.**

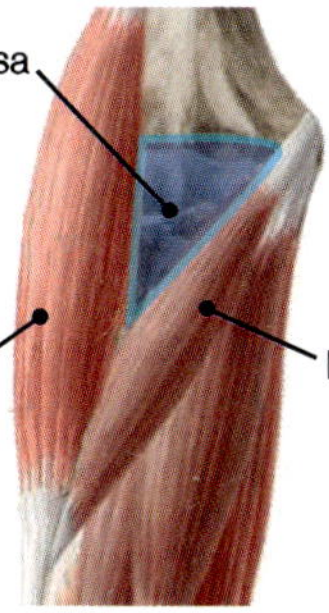

Fig 7.67 The cubital fossa and it's borders.

The carpal tunnel

As described in the learning notes on page 134:
"The carpal tunnel is a narrow canal found on the palmar side of the hand where the four tendons of the **flexor digitorum profundus**, the four tendons of the **flexor digitorum superficialis**, the tendon of the **flexor pollicis longus**, and the **median nerve** pass through from the forearm into the hand. The tunnel is formed by the carpal bones and a strong fibrous band, known as the **flexor retinaculum**, which arches over them. The flexor retinaculum attaches to the scaphoid and trapezium bones on the radial side, and the pisiform and the hook of Hamate on the ulnar side of the hand.

A common medical condition of note is carpal tunnel syndrome (CTS), which arises when one or more of the nine flexor tendons swells and further narrows the canal, resulting in the entrapment and compression of the median nerve."

The snuffbox

The anatomical snuffbox, also known as the radial fossa, is a depression located on the lateral dorsal aspect of the hand, at the level of the carpal bones, which you can visualize when the thumb is extended.

The borders of the anatomical snuff box are the tendon of the **extensor pollicis longus** (medial border), **tendons of the abductor pollicis longus** and **extensor pollicis brevis** (lateral border), **styloid process of the radius** (proximal border), and **the scaphoid and trapezium** (floor).

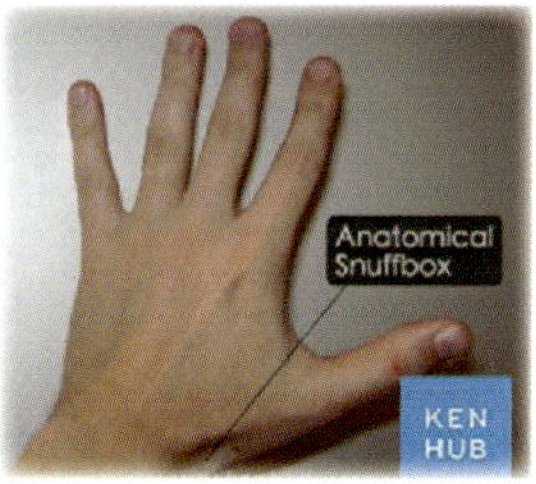

Fig 7.68 The anatomical snuffbox.

It contains the **radial artery**, the **superficial branch of the radial nerve**, and the **cephalic vein**.

The clinical significance of the anatomical significance is seen in the event of a fall on the outstretched hand.[75] A fracture of the scaphoid would disrupt its blood supply leading to avascular necrosis.[76]

The Anatomy and Examinations of the Lower Limb

By Robert Vardanyan

Again, I regret the immense amount of anatomy within this chapter, but to quote Lao Tzu a second time in this book - "*A journey of a thousand miles must begin with a single step*". Without a doubt, he was trying to convey that you must follow the natural order of learning the anatomy of the lower limbs first before progressing on to the testing of said anatomy. And so I have structured this chapter in the same way as the upper limbs before it; bones and joints, muscles, and testing, nerves, arteries, veins, and lastly, relevant anatomical structures. I have also added an asterisk to vital muscles within the lower limb station.
Also, note that when we discuss the 'leg', we are referring to the area between the knee and the ankle, and not the lower limb as a whole.

1 Identify the bones and joints of the lower limb

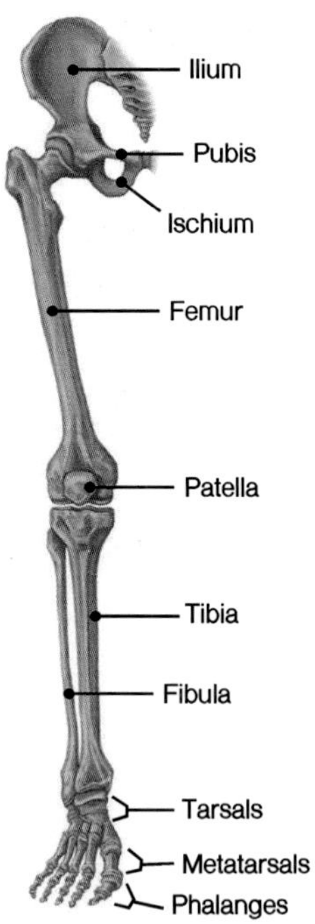

Fig 8.1 The bones of the lower limb.

In some circles, the pelvic bone (or aspects of it) are considered to be the most proximal beginnings of the lower limb, but we will begin our discussion from the **hip joint**, which is a ball and socket synovial joint formed from the articulation of the acetabulum and femoral head.[33]

The **acetabulum**, as you may know, is a deep hemispherical concavity covered in articular cartilage within the pelvic bone. It is further specialised through a fibrocartilaginous collar known as the acetabular labrum, which deepens the depression at the hip joint.

The hip joint is a vital weight-bearing joint, that through its many ligaments and surrounding muscles is actually very stable. However, the stability of this ball and socket joint comes at the price of a large range of motion, although this is certainly defied by many people within the acrobatics and martial arts community.[77]

The five ligaments of the hip joint begin with the **ligament of the femoral head**. This is an intracapsular ligament that literally attaches the femur to the acetabulum inside of the joint. The four remaining ligaments are the **transverse acetabular ligament** (which stems from the acetabular labrum) and the three extracapsular ligaments (in that they attach around the capsule of the synovial joint). These are the **iliofemoral**, **pubofemoral**, and **ischiofemoral** ligaments, all appropriately named based upon their origins and insertions. The iliofemoral ligament is also what limits the extension of the hip joint.[78]

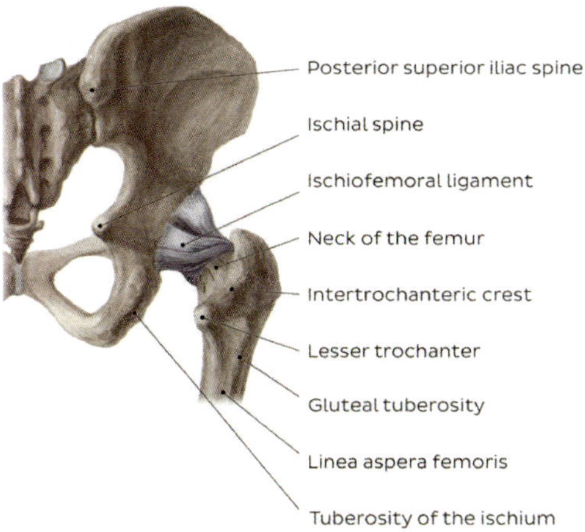

Fig 8.2 The ligaments, bones, and respective surface landmarks of the hip joint, pelvis, and femur, viewed posteriorly.

Fig 8.3 The ligaments, bones, and respective surface landmarks of the hip joint, pelvis, and femur, viewed anteriorly.

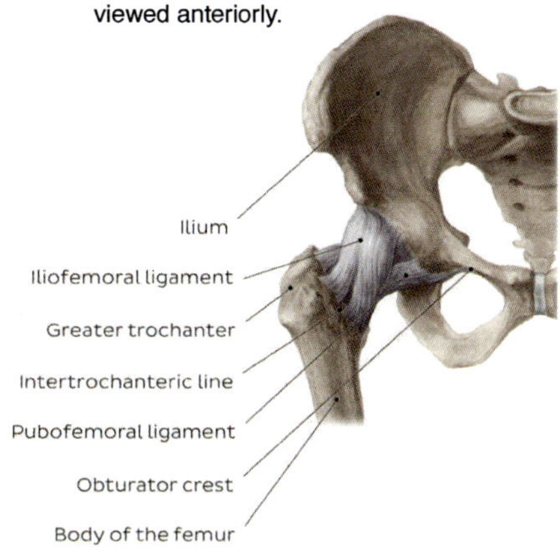

External rotation[33] | **Internal rotation**[33] | **Adduction**[33] | **Abduction**[33]

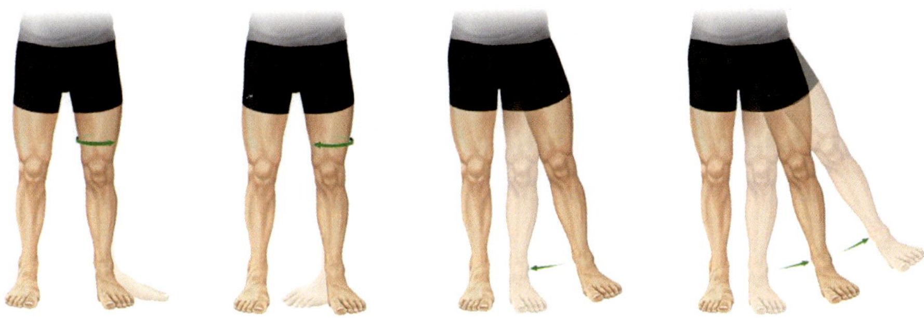

External rotation[33]: Obturator internus, Obturator externus, Superior gemellus, Inferior gemellus, Quadratus femoris, Piriformis

Internal rotation[33]: Gluteus medius, Gluteus minimus

Adduction[33]: Adductor longus, Adductor brevis, Adductor magnus, Pectineus, Gracilis, Quadratus femoris

Abduction[33]: Gluteus medius, Gluteus minimus, Piriformis

Extension[33] | **Flexion**[33]

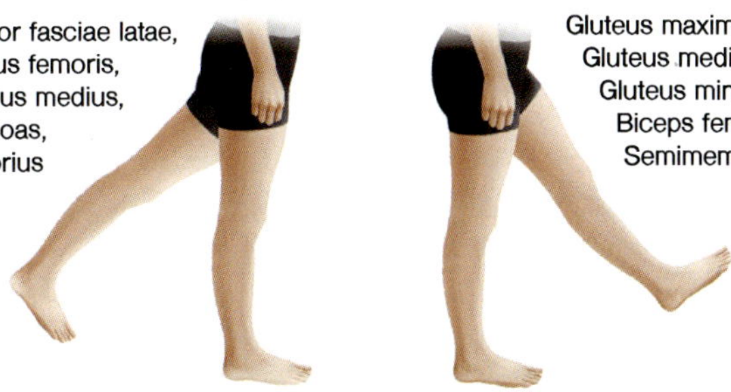

Tensor fasciae latae, Rectus femoris, Gluteus medius, Iliopsoas, Sartorius

Gluteus maximus, Gluteus medius, Gluteus minimus, Biceps femoris, Semimembranosus

Fig 8.4 The movements at the hip joint and the muscles that initiate those motions. Circumduction has not been included, but it is a culmination of the efforts of all the mentioned muscles.

Femur

The femur is the long bone of the thigh that proximally articulates with the **acetabulum** to form the **hip joint**, and distally it articulates with the **tibia** and the **patella** to form the **knee joint**.

Of clinical importance is also the neck of the femur, which, angled at 126° to the femoral shaft, increases the range of motion of the hip joint but is very prone to fractures, especially amongst older people with osteoporosis.[79]

Of importance in the OSPE is also the **greater trochanter** and the **lesser trochanter**, as labelled in **Fig 8.2** & **8.3**. The greater trochanter is a large palpable projection that is an insertion point for the **gluteus medius, gluteus minimus, piriformis, obturator internus, superior gemellus, inferior gemellus and obturator externus muscles**. It is found laterally and at the level of the femoral head.[33] The lesser trochanter is the projection that is the attachment site for **iliopsoas** and part of the **adductor magnus** muscles.

As the neck of the femur leads on to the shaft, three roughened descending ridges merge to form the linea aspera. The **gluteal tuberosity** (lateral ridge) provides an attachment site for the deep, distal fibres of the **gluteus maximus** muscle; the **pectineal line** (intermediate ridge) gives attachment to the **pectineus**; and the **intertrochanteric line** (medial ridge) is the origin of the **vastus medialis** muscle. Within the ridges, numerous other muscles are also inserted.

Distally, the **lateral and medial condyles** of the femur project to form the **tibiofemoral articulation** and the patellar surface articulates with the patella at the **patellofemoral articulation** of the knee joint. This is a synovial hinge joint which permits **flexion** and **extension** of the leg.

Between the significantly incompatible tibiofemoral articulation, sit the **medial and lateral menisci**. These are fibrocartilaginous pads which increase joint stability and absorb shock by dissipating pressure amongst a greater surface area.

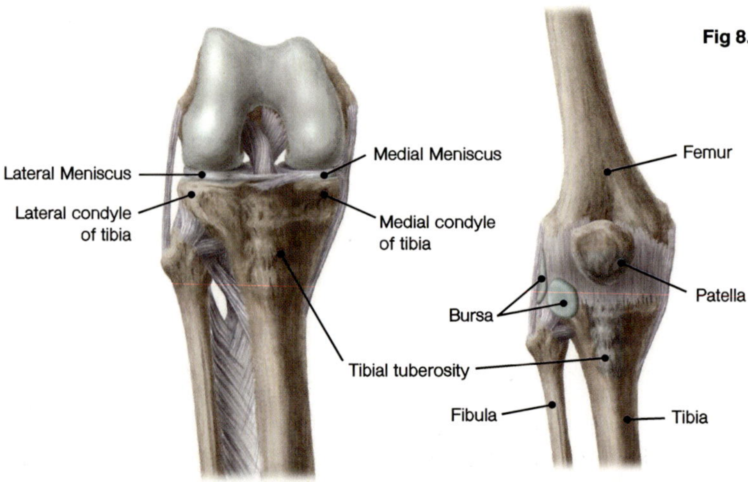

Fig 8.5 The ligaments, bones, and respective surface landmarks of the knee joint.

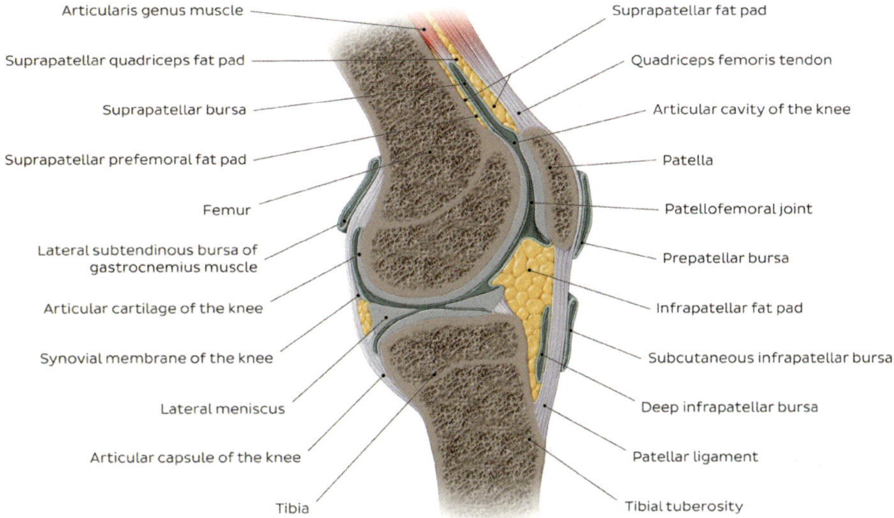

Fig 8.6 Sagittal view of the knee joint.

Patella

The patella is the largest **sesamoid bone** in the body, and it resides in the **quadriceps femoris tendon**.[33] It provides a fulcrum (leverage point) to increase the efficacy of this most powerful group of knee extensors and serves to protect the knee joint from trauma anteriorly.

Four synovial-filled sacs, known as **bursae**, can also be found in the knee joint – the suprapatellar, the prepatellar, the infrapatellar, and the semimembranosus bursa – along with **collateral ligaments** that attach to femoral epicondyles on either side of the knee joint – the tibial (medial) collateral ligament and the fibular (lateral) collateral ligament – and the tibia and fibula respectively, to stabilise the hinge motion of the knee.[80]

Learning notes

When the knee is flexed, it also has a very small degree of medial and lateral rotation. This is produced by the biceps femoris (lateral rotation) and semimembranosus, semitendinosus, gracilis, sartorius and popliteus (medial rotation).

Fig 8.7 The main movements of the knee joint.

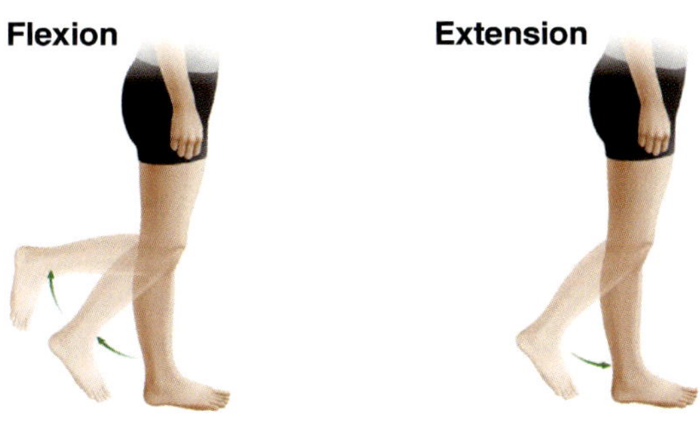

Flexion: Produced by the hamstrings, gracilis, sartorius and popliteus.

Extension: Produced by the quadriceps femoris, which inserts into the tibial tuberosity.

Fig 8.8 The bones of the leg.

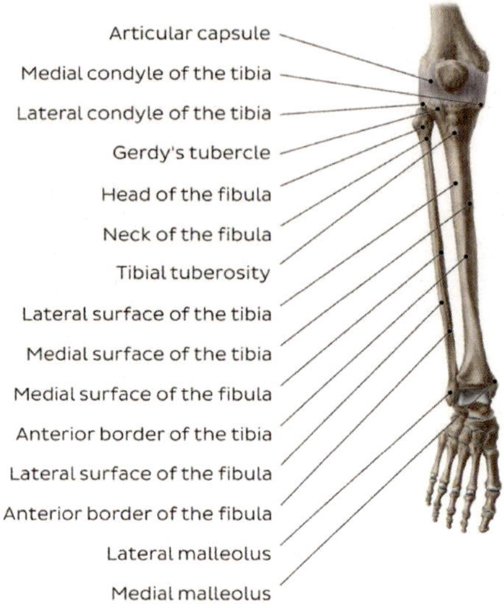

Tibia

The tibia is the main weight-bearing bone of the leg which articulates with the femur at the **tibiofemoral articulation** of the knee, the fibula at the **superior and inferior tibiofibular joints**, and the talus at the **talocrural joint** of the ankle, where it forms the **medial malleolus** (the bony projection felt medially at the ankle).[81]

Fibula

The fibula is located laterally to the tibia, and it is not a weight-bearing bone. Instead, it is an attachment site for numerous tendons and it forms the **lateral malleolus** (bony projection felt laterally at the ankle) at the **talocrural joint**.[81]
As mentioned, it articulates with the tibia at two **tibiofibular joints**, proximally and distally.
Note that it does not articulate with the femur.

The **talocrural joint** is a synovial hinge joint formed between the **medial malleolus of the tibia**, the **lateral malleolus of the fibula** (which join together to form a socket), and the **talus bone** of the foot, which is one of seven tarsus bones. This bone then articulates with the **calcaneus** (another tarsus bone) to form the **talocalcaneal joint**. Alongside the inferior tibiofibular joint, these two joints form the ankle.

The talocrural joint allows for dorsiflexion and plantarflexion of the foot, and the talocalcaneal joint allows for a small degree of foot inversion and eversion.

Plantar flexion | **Dorsiflexion**

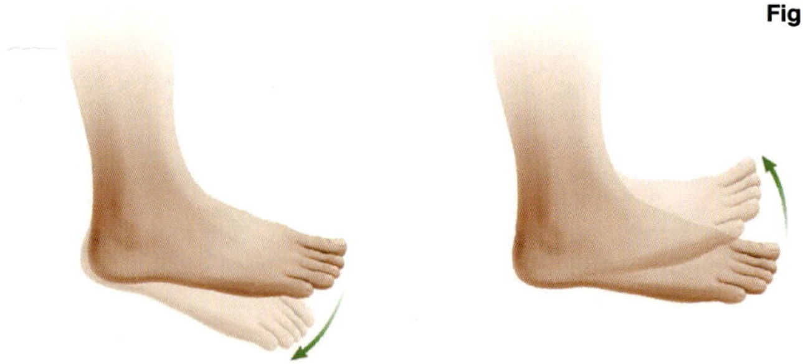

Fig 8.9 The movements of the foot at the talocrural joint of the ankle. Plantar flexion can be thought of as planting your foot onto the ground to help you remember.

Produced by the muscles in the posterior compartment of the leg (gastrocnemius, soleus, plantaris and posterior tibialis)

Produced by the muscles in the anterior compartment of the leg (tibialis anterior, extensor hallucis longus and extensor digitorum

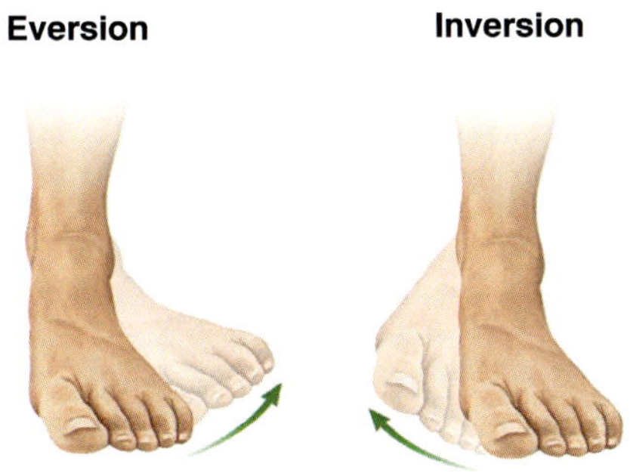

Fig 8.10 The movements of the foot at the talocalcaneonavicular joint of the ankle.

Much like the bony anatomy of the hand, the foot is formed from five groups of bones; **the tarsals**; **the metatarsals**; and **the proximal**, **intermediate**, and **distal phalanges**.

Tarsals

The **talus** is an irregularly shaped proximal bone which forms the link between the foot and the leg through the talocrural joint. It then articulates with the calcaneus at the subtalar (talocalcaneal) joint and the **navicular** bone at the talonavicular joint to form the **talocalcaneonavicular joint**, which is important in the eversion and inversion of the foot, as pictured in **Fig 8.10**.[82]

The calcaneus is the largest bone in the foot and it lies below the talus to form the heel of the foot. It is vital in taking the weight of the body and is attached to the **Achilles tendon**.[33]

The talus and calcaneus constitute the proximal row of the tarsal bones, whereas the navicular bone constitutes the intermediate row. It articulates with the three **cuneiform bones**, which in turn articulate with the three medial **metatarsal bones** and the **cuboid**. The cuboid is the main bone of the midfoot, and it sits in the distal row of the tarsals alongside the cuneiforms and articulates with the lateral two metatarsals distally and the calcaneus proximally.

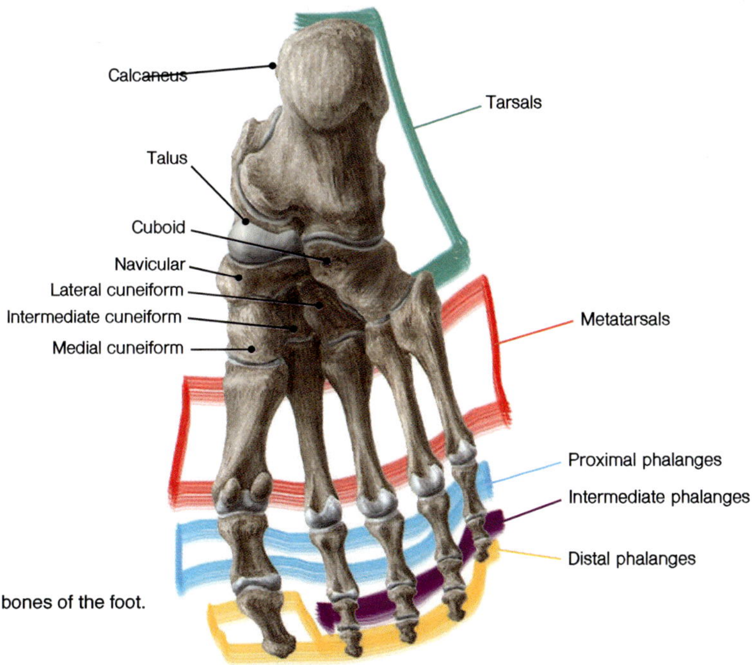

Fig 8.11 The bones of the foot.

Alongside the metatarsals, the tarsals are essential in forming the arches of the foot, comprised of the medial **longitudinal arch**, the **lateral longitudinal arch**, and the **transverse arch**. These are important in lower limb mobility.[83]

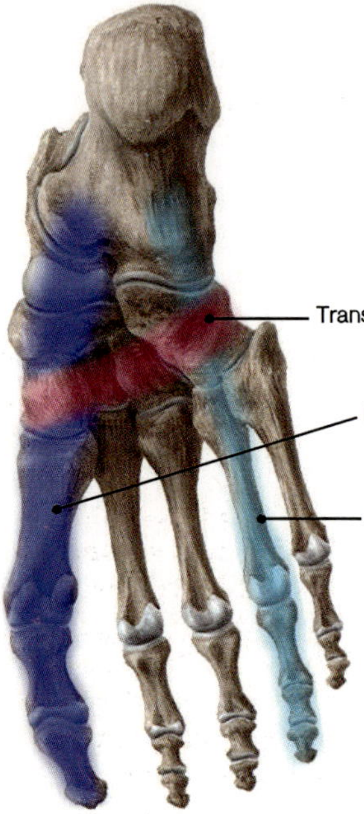

Fig 8.12 The arches of the foot.

The five metatarsals, connected to the tarsals proximally, have articulations with the five **proximal phalanges of the foot**, forming the **metatarsophalangeal** joints. The movements permitted in the **metatarsophalangeal** joints are flexion, extension, abduction, adduction, and circumduction.

The distal phalanges then form the most distal aspects of the foot. Each digit of the foot, much like in the hand, has three phalanges – the proximal, intermediate, and distal.
However, the first digit of the foot, known as the **hallux** (or big toe) only has two phalanges – the proximal and distal – and therefore only has one **interphalangeal joint**. These joints, much like in the hands, only allow flexion and extension.

2 Muscles of the lower limb

The muscles that act upon the lower limb are numerous in number and diverse in function. Therefore, we will discuss the muscles by categorising them into eight different groups based upon anatomical location. These groups are:

1) Superficial muscles of the pelvic girdle
2) Deep muscles of the pelvic girdle
3) Anterior compartment of the thigh
4) Medial compartment of the thigh
5) Posterior compartment of the thigh
6) Anterior compartment of leg
7) Posterior compartment of leg
8) Lateral compartment of leg

Within each of these groups we will discuss the functions of the muscles, relevant tendons and joints, the appropriate clinical examinations, and brief neurovasculature. Please keep in mind that neurovasculature will be appropriately explored in later learning objectives.
Furthermore, we will delve deeper into only some of the muscles listed, as this is what is required within the OSPEs. **These key muscles will be marked with an asterisk.**
The intrinsic muscles of the foot will not be discussed, as they are not required in the OSPE.

1) The superficial muscles of the pelvic girdle

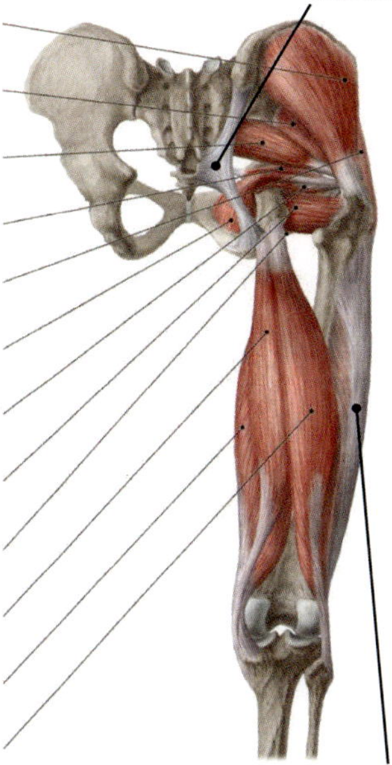

Fig 8.13 The relevant muscles, tendons, and ligaments of the pelvis and femur.

The key muscles of interest are the pectoralis major and the **gluteus maximus**, **gluteus medius**, **gluteus minimus**, and **tensor fascia latae**.

Gluteus maximus*

The gluteus maximus is the largest and most superficial of the gluteal muscles, and it is the **main extensor of the thigh** and it assists in **lateral rotation**. The gluteus maximus originates from the **sacrum, ilium, thoracolumbar fascia, and the sacrotuberous ligament** (labelled in **Fig 8.13**), and it descends to insert at the **gluteal tuberosity of the femur** and the **iliotibial tract** (which is a strong longitudinal fibrous reinforcement of the fascia lata that inserts at the lateral condyle of the tibia).

The innervation is supplied by the **inferior gluteal nerve**.[33]

It is not expected for you to test the function of the gluteus maximus in the OSPE, but for reference, the testing of the muscle involves asking the patient to extend their thigh against resistance provided by you, the examiner, whilst they are lying on their abdomen. Palpation is also required of the gluteus maximus when testing it's function.

Gluteus medius* and gluteus minimus*

The **gluteus medius** and **minimus** muscles, also referred to as the small gluteal muscles, are found in the posterior pelvis, travelling from the **ilium to the femur**.

The gluteus medius muscle lies in the intermediate layer of the gluteal muscles, between the gluteus maximus and minimus. It works synergistically with the gluteus minimus (known together as the small gluteal muscles) to **abduct and medially rotate** the thigh, as their points of origin and insertion are so very close. The gluteus medius originates from the **gluteal surface of the ilium** and inserts into the lateral surface of the **greater trochanter**, whilst the gluteus minimus, which is also fan-shaped, originates just inferiorly and deep to gluteus medius on the ileum and inserts at the anterior aspect of the greater trochanter. Note also that the gluteus medius and the gluteus minimus have a fundamental role in stabilising the pelvis, together, they share vasculature and innervation from the **superior gluteal nerve**.

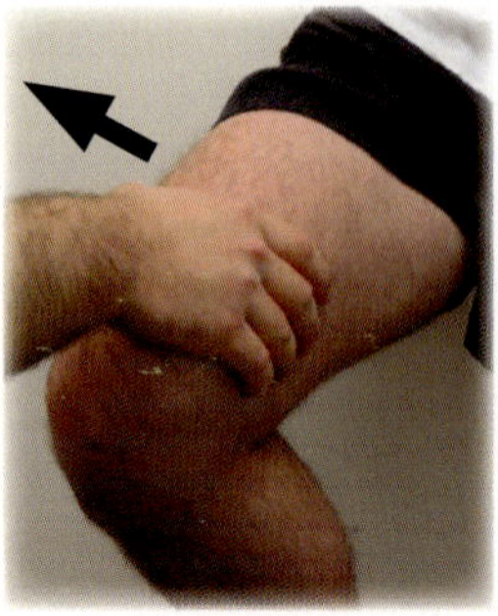

Fig 8.14 The abduction test for the gluteus medius and the gluteus minimus.

To assess the function of the small gluteal muscles, specifically, the gluteus medius, ask the patient to **abduct their thigh** against resistance whilst lying down on their side. You, as the examiner, should provide resistance to the abducting motion and palpate the gluteus medius. It is also acceptable to perform this test with the patient sitting on the end of the bed.

To request this test from the patient ask them:
"Can you bend your knees and bring your thighs away from each other, against resistance?"

Trendelenburg sign (required)

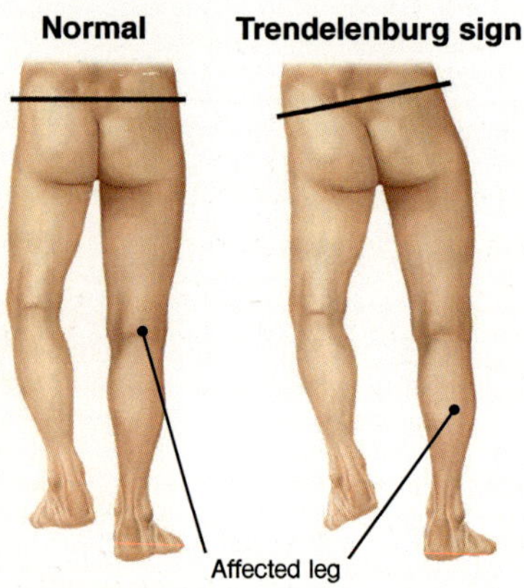

Fig 8.15 The Trendelenburg sign.

The Trendelenburg sign is the result of **weakness of the hip abductor muscles**, specifically the gluteus medius and the gluteus minimus (which, as mentioned, work to stabilise the pelvis during movement). This stems from **damage to the superior gluteal nerve**, which innervates these small gluteal muscles.
Patient's with the Trendelenburg sign present with a dropping of the pelvis **opposite to the affected side, when they stand on the affected leg.**

Tensor fascia latae*

The final superficial muscle of the gluteal region is the tensor fascia latae (labelled in **Fig 8.16**), which works synergistically with the small gluteal muscles to **abduct and medially rotate the thigh** and assist the gluteus maximus through stabilising the thigh when extended. It originates from the **anterior superior iliac spine** and inserts into the **iliotibial tract** like some fibres of the gluteus maximus. It is also innervated by the **superior gluteal nerve**.

2) The deep muscles of the pelvic girdle

The deep muscles of the pelvic girdle work to laterally r**otate and weakly abduct the thigh**, and **stabilise the femoral head within the acetabulum**. These muscles are the **piriformis**, **obturator internus**, the **superior and inferior gamelli**, and the **quadratus femoris** (which should not be confused with the quadriceps femoris group of muscles). For the OSPE, this is the knowledge required about the deep muscles of the pelvic girdle.

3) Anterior compartment of the thigh

The thigh is divided into three muscular compartments: the anterior compartment, medial compartment and the posterior compartment.

The muscles in the anterior compartment of the thigh are the **quadriceps femoris**, **sartorius**, **pectineus**, and the **iliopsoas**, and they are all innervated by the **femoral nerve.**

Fig 8.16 The muscles of the anterior compartment of the thigh.

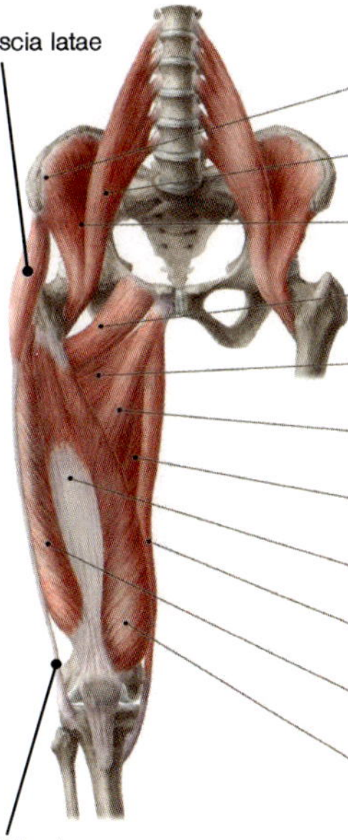

Iliopsoas*

The iliopsoas stems from the merging of the **psoas major and iliacus**, which come together to form the tendon that attaches to the **lesser trochanter** of the femur. It assists in the **flexion and lateral rotation of the thigh**.

Sartorius*

The sartorius is a superficial long muscle that originates from the **anterior superior iliac spine** and traverses down the entire femur to attach to the **medial surface of the tibia**. It is the longest muscle of the body and it assists at **flexion, lateral rotation, and weak abduction of the thigh**. It also assists in medial rotation of the leg when the knee joint is flexed.

Pectineus

It originates from the pectineal line on the anterior surface of the pelvic bone, and attaches to the pectineal line on the posterior side of the femur, just inferior to the lesser trochanter. It assists in the **adduction and flexion of the hip joint**.

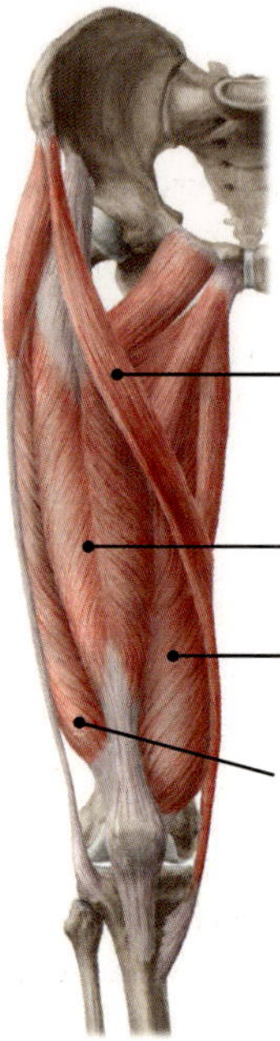

Fig 8.17 The quadriceps femoris group of muscles.

Quadriceps femoris*

The quadriceps femoris is a large and powerful **muscle group** of the thigh that constitutes four individual muscles- the **vastus medialis, vastus intermedius, vastus lateralis,** and the **rectus femoris**.
It functions to cause **flexion at the hip joint and extension at the knee joint** through its attachment to the **patella** (which is a sesamoid bone residing in the patellar ligament).
The vastus lateralis originates from the greater trochanter and the lateral lip of linea aspera, the vastus intermedius originates from the anterior and lateral surfaces of the femoral shaft, the vastus medialis originates from the intertrochanteric line and medial lip of the linea aspera, and the rectus femoris originates from the supra-acetabular groove. These four muscles merge to form the **quadriceps femoris tendon** which becomes the patellar ligament at the patella and inserts into the **tuberosity of the tibia**.

To assess the function of the quadriceps, ask the patient to **extend their leg** whilst sitting on the edge of the bed. As the examiner, you should apply firm resistance to the distal part of the leg and palpate the contraction of the quadriceps at the anterior surface of their thigh.
This is pictured in **Fig 8.18**.

To request this test from the patient ask:
"Can you kick your leg out for me whilst I try to resist you?"

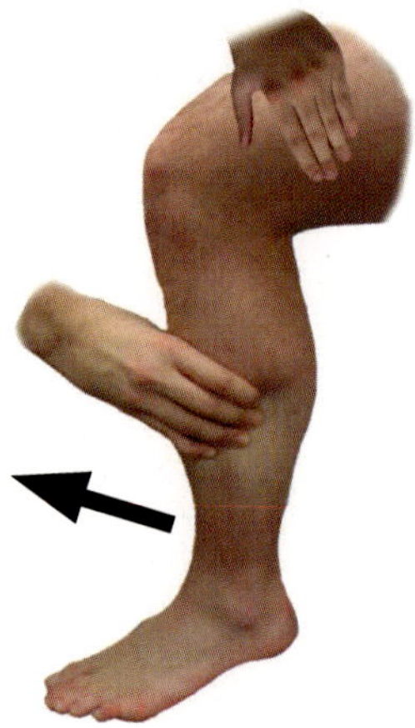

Fig 8.18 The leg extension test for the quadriceps femoris.

4) Medial compartment of the thigh

The muscles in the medial compartment of the thigh are the **gracilis**, **obturator externus**, **adductor brevis**, **adductor longus** and **adductor magnus**, and they are known as the hip abductors (pictured in **Fig 8.16**).[33]
Also, they are all innervated by the **obturator nerve** and supplied by the **obturator artery**.

Gracilis

The gracilis is the most superficial and medial of the hip adductors, originating from the inferior rami of the pubis and inserting into the medial surface of the tibia. It is involved in the **adduction of the thigh and flexion of the leg**.

Obturator externus

The obturator externus originates from the membrane of the obturator foramen, pass under the neck of the femur, and inserts at the posterior aspect of the greater trochanter. It is involved in the **adduction and lateral rotation of the thigh**.

Adductor longus, brevis, and magnus*

The adductor longus is the most anterior of the remaining three hip adductors and it forms the medial border of the femoral triangle. It originates from the **pubis** and inserts at **linea aspera of the femur**.

The adductor brevis is a short muscle, lying underneath the adductor longus, and it originates from the body of the **pubis and inferior pubic rami** and also attaches to the **linea aspera**.

The adductor magnus is the largest muscle in the medial compartment and it lies posteriorly to the other adductor muscles. It has two parts which function to **adduct the thigh**, but can then either cause flexion or extension depending on which aspect of the adductor magnus is contracted. These two parts are called the **adductor part** and the **hamstring part**, and this is actually very relevant to you as we will be discussing the different innervations of these two parts in the nervous supply to the lower limb learning objective.

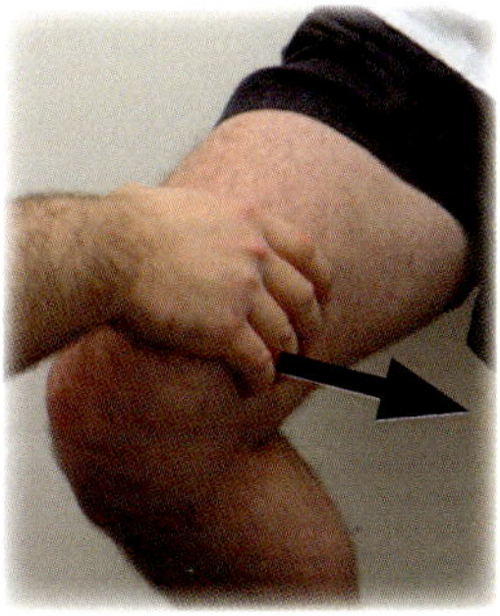

To assess the function of the hip adductors, ask the patient to **adduct their thigh** whilst the patient is sitting on the edge of the bed. As the examiner, you should apply firm resistance to the distal part of their thigh and palpate the contraction of the hip adductors at the superior medial surface of their thigh. This is pictured in **Fig 8.19**.

To request this test from the patient ask them to:
"Can you bend your knees and bring your legs together?"

Fig 8.19 The hip adduction test for the muscles of the medial compartment of the thigh.

5) Posterior compartment of the thigh

The muscles in the posterior compartment of the thigh include the **biceps femoris**, **semitendinosus** and **semimembranosus**, and they are known as the hamstrings.[33] They are pictured in **Fig 8.13**.

All three of these muscles cross the hip joint and knee joint, and therefore have functions at both of these joints. Their principal action is to **extend the thigh** at the hip joint and **flex the leg** at the knee joint. When the knee is in the flexed position, the biceps femoris can then externally rotate the leg whereas the semimembranosus and semitendinosus can act as internal rotators at the knee joint.

Biceps femoris*

Much like the biceps brachii in the arm, the biceps femoris muscle has two heads and is named appropriately. The long head of the biceps femoris originates from the ischial tuberosity through a shared tendon with the semitendinosus and the short head originates from the linea aspera. Both heads then unite to form the biceps femoris tendon to insert into the head of the fibula. Alongside the extension of the thigh at the hip joint, the biceps femoris also functions in the lateral rotation of the leg when the knee is flexed.

Semitendinosus*

The semitendinosus is named as such because of it significantly longer tendon when inserting into the medial surface of the tibia, behind then tendon attachment of the gracilis. It originates from the same tendon as the long head of the biceps femoris at the ischial tuberosity, and other than extension of the thigh at the hip joint, it functions in the medial rotation of the leg when the knee joint is flexed alongside the semimembranosus.

Semimemranosus*

The semimembranosus muscle also originates from the ischial tuberosity like the biceps femoris and the semitendinosus, but it arises more superiorly to the proximal tendon of the aforementioned muscles. It then inserts at the medial condyle of the tibia, where it functions to extend the thigh and medially rotate the leg when flexed at the knee joint.

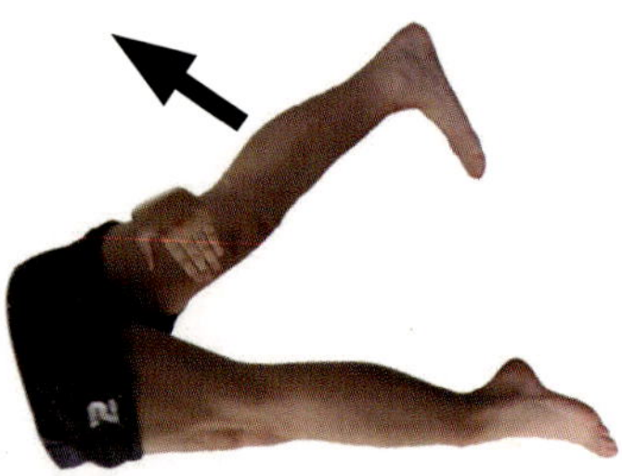

Fig 8.20 The thigh extension test to assess the hamstrings.

To assess the function of the hamstrings, ask the patient to extend their thigh while they lie prone on the bed.
As the examiner, you should apply firm resistance to their thigh and palpate the contraction of the hamstrings at the posterior surface of their thigh.
This is pictured in **Fig 8.20**, and is not an examination you are expected to perfom during the OSPE.

To request this test from the patient ask them to:
"Can you lie flat on your stomach and rise your leg whilst I resist you?"

6) Anterior compartment of the leg

There are three main muscles in the anterior compartment of the leg are the **tibialis anterior**, **extensor digitorum longus**, and **extensor hallucis longus**.[33]
Collectively, they act to dorsiflex and invert the foot at the ankle joint, which are required when standing on your toes. As is in the name, the extensor digitorum longus and extensor hallucis longus also extend the toes, and the muscles of this compartment are innervated by the **deep fibular nerve** (L4-L5), and blood is supplied via the **anterior tibial artery**.

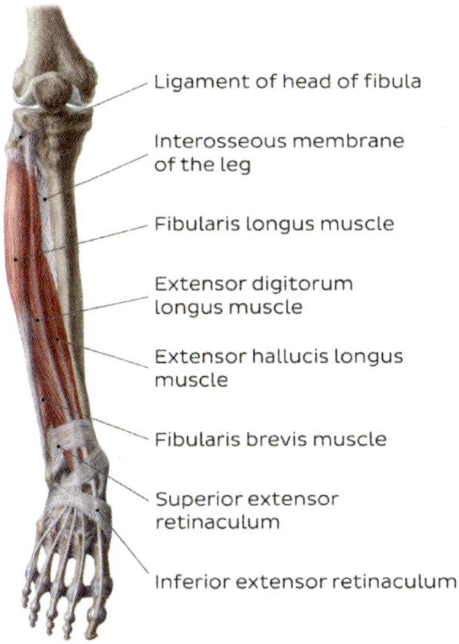

Fig 8.21 The muscles of the anterior and lateral compartments of the leg.

Tibialis anterior*

The tibialis anterior muscle is the largest and most superficial of the anterior muscles, and it originates and descends from the **lateral surface of the tibia**. It then inserts into the plantar side of the **medial cuneiform and base of the first metatarsal bone**, where it is the strongest **dorsiflexor of the foot**. It also functions in the inversion of the foot.

Extensor digitorum longus

The EDL originates at the lateral tibial condyle and the medial surface of the fibula where it then descends down to form four tendons which insert at the intermediate and distal phalanges of the four lateral digits. of the four lesser toes. These tendons can be easily palpated upon the extension of the four lateral digits and dorsiflexion of the foot.

Extensor hallucis longus

The EHL has its origin at the medial side of the fibula and interosseous membrane, and it is located deep to the EDL and the tibialis anterior. It's tendon then inserts at the distal phalanx of the hallux, and causes extension of this digit along with dorsiflexion of the foot.

To test the power of these muscles, ask the patient to stand on their heels, which causes them to dorsiflex their feet. If the patient is lying down, you can ask them to their ankles such that their toes face the ceiling.
In fact, this is more preferable, as it will be easier for you to stabilise the ankle joint and provide effective resistance to the dorsiflexion.

Dorsiflexion

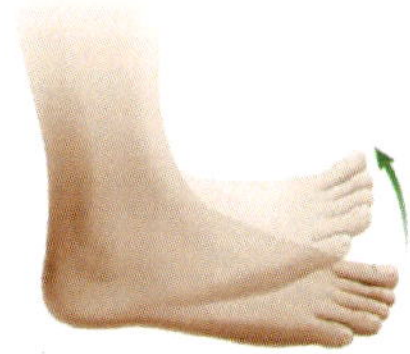

Fig 8.22 The test to assess the muscles of the anterior compartment of the leg.

7) Posterior compartment of the leg

The posterior leg is the largest of the three compartments, and the muscles in this area work on **plantar flexion of the foot**. They are innervated by the **tibial nerve**, a terminal branch of the sciatic nerve. We will discuss these muscles by dividing them into two categories; superficial and deep. This is to match the knowledge required in the OSPE surrounding this compartment.

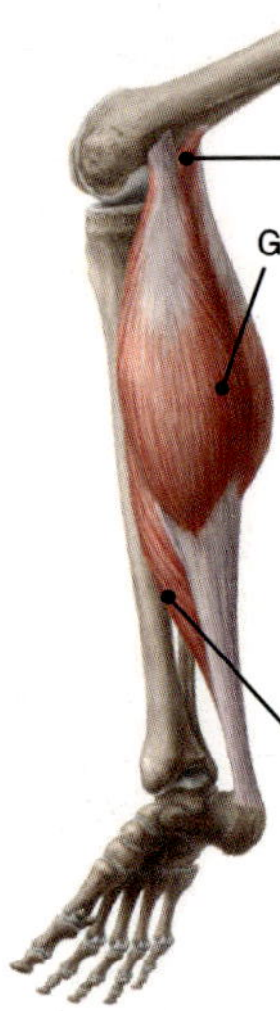

Fig 8.23 The superficial muscles of the posterior leg compartment.

Superficial muscles of the posterior compartment*

There are three superficial muscles and they combine together to form a single tendon that inserts into the calcaneus of the foot (the heel bone), known as the **calcaneal (Achilles) tendon**.

The **gastrocnemius** has a medial and lateral head, and it is the most superficial of all the muscles in the posterior leg.
The lateral head originates from the **lateral femoral condyle**, and the medial head originates from the **medial femoral condyle**.
The fibres then converge to form the gastrocnemius muscle belly, which further combines distally in the leg with the soleus and the very thin tendon from the plantaris to form the calcaneal tendon, which inserts into the calcaneus. However, due to it's attachment to the femur, it also works in the **flexion of the knee joint**.

The plantaris is a relatively small muscle which arises from the femur (superior to the gastrocnemius), while the soleus originates from the fibular head and the medial aspect of the tibia. Both these muscles form tendons that combine to form the Achilles tendon, which then **plantarflexes the foot** at the ankle joint.

To test these muscles, ask the patient to point their toes away from themselves by bend their ankle like they would when firmly pressing a pedal.

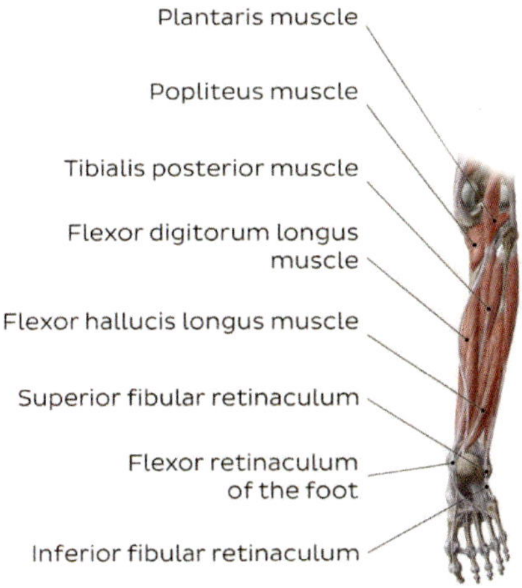

Fig 8.24 The deep muscles of the posterior leg compartment.

Deep muscles of the posterior compartment
There are four muscles in the deep compartment of the posterior leg.

The **popliteus** is the most superior of which and it acts to **rotate the femur on the tibia**.
The **tibialis posterior** then **inverts and plantarflexes the foot**, whilst the **flexor hallucis longus** and **flexor digitorum longus** work on the **flexion of the hallux and the lateral four digits**, respectively.

Inversion of the foot is pictured in **Fig 8.10**.

8) Lateral compartment of the leg

The lateral compartment of the leg consists of the **fibularis longus** and the **fibularis brevis**, as pictured in **Fig 8.21**. The fibularis brevis is shorter than the fibularis longus, as the name suggests, and both muscles are innervated by the **peroneal nerve** and **work on eversion of the foot (Fig 8.10)**. The fibularis longus also assists in the plantarflexion of the foot.

As mentioned, the required knowledge of the muscles of the foot is minimal in the OSPE, and whilst I strongly advise that you consider the muscles of the foot as it's own separate muscle category in your anatomy revision of the lower limb, we will not be discussing it in this OSPE book anymore than the generous diagram below provided by the team at Kenhub.

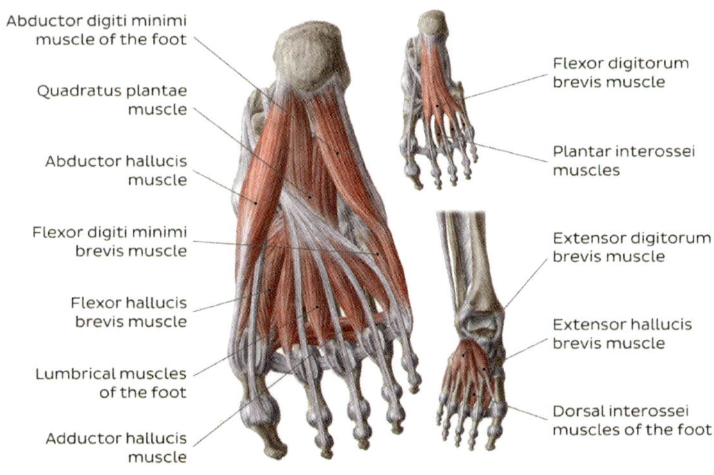

Fig 8.25 The intrinsic muscles of the foot.

3 The nerve supply to the lower limb

The nerves of the lower limb originate from the lumbar (L1-L4) and sacral plexuses (L4-S4) in the pelvis. They key nerves of interest for the OSPEs are the sciatic, gluteal, femoral, obturator, and the superficial and deep peroneal nerves. These are major peripheral nerves of the lower limb, and be aware not to confuse the peroneal nerves with the perineal nerve (which supplies the pudendal nerve of the perineal area). The tibial nerve, which is one of the two terminal branches of the sciatic nerve, is also a very clinically significant nerve, but knowledge of the nerve and it's testing is minimally required for the OSPE. Although, rather contradictorily, familiarity with the popliteal fossa and the ankle jerk reflex, produced by the gastrocnemius and soleus muscles which are innervated by the tibial nerve, is a key skill required for the exam.

Also, we will discuss each key nerve individually and the motor component examination of each, and then we will discuss the sensation of the lower limb in general.

Sciatic nerve

The sciatic nerve is the longest nerve in the body, and stems from the anterior and posterior divisions of nerve roots L4, L5, S1, S2, and S3. It leaves the pelvic cavity through the greater sciatic foramen and it comes out deep to the inferior border of the piriformis.

To path the anatomical course for the sciatic nerve within the OSPE, palpate for the posterior superior iliac spine, the ischial tuberosity, and the greater trochanter of the femur. The sciatic nerve leaves the greater sciatic foramen and enters the gluteal region midway between the PSIS and ischial tuberosity and travels down half way between the ischial tuberosity and the greater trochanter. Therefore, you can path the nerve as a curve between the midpoint of the PSIS and ischial tuberosity and the midpoint between the greater trochanter and the ischial tuberosity upon its entry into the gluteal region.

It then travels deep to the long head of the biceps femoris and terminates at the popliteal fossa, forming the tibial and common fibular nerve. This is one straight long line to the popliteal fossa.
It is vital to know how to surface mark the sciatic nerve in the OSPE.

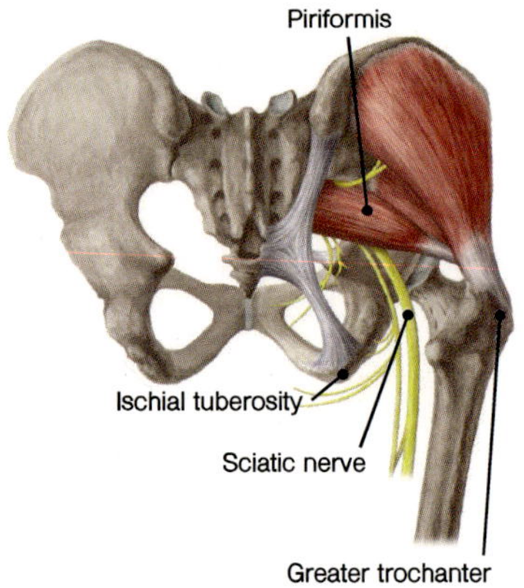

Fig 8.26 The sciatic nerve.

The sciatic nerve directly innervates the hamstrings (posterior thigh compartment) and the hamstring portion of the adductor magnus. However, if we were to consider its indirect innervation through its two terminal branches, then it also innervates the entirety of the leg and foot. Directly, the sciatic nerve does not have a sensory function in the thigh, but again, considering it's two terminal branches, it indirectly provides sensory innervation to the entirety of the leg and foot. The common fibular branch will be discussed in more detail when discussing the superior and deep peroneal nerves.

Therefore, to test the sciatic nerve, ask the patient to flex their knee joint. This must be done with resistance as even when testing nerves, resistance is essential, and it can be done while the patient is lying on their back or their front.

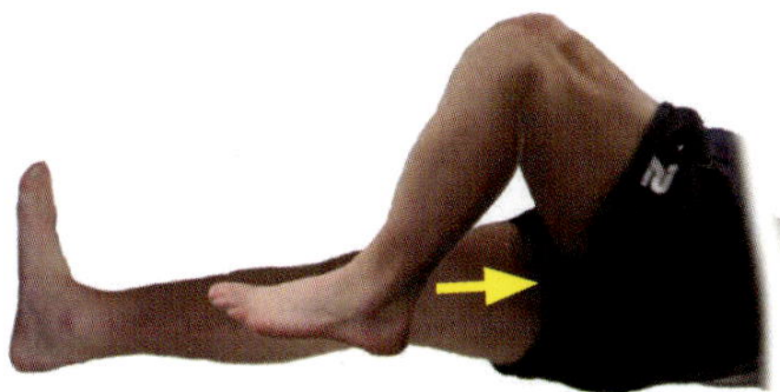

Fig 8.27 The knee flexion test for the sciatic nerve.

To request this test from the patient ask them to:
"Can you bend your knee and bring your leg to your buttocks while I apply some resistance?"

Gluteal nerve

The nerves that supply the gluteal region are the superior and inferior gluteal nerves.
The superior gluteal nerve arises from nerve roots L4, L5, and S1, and it enters the gluteal region through the sciatic foramen superior to the piriformis, where it travels to innervate the gluteus medius, the gluteus minimus, the tensor fascia latae, and the piriformis. Damage to the superior gluteal nerve can result in the aforementioned Trendelenburg gait.
The inferior gluteal nerve stems from nerve roots L5, S1, and S2, and it travels to innervate the gluteus maximus.

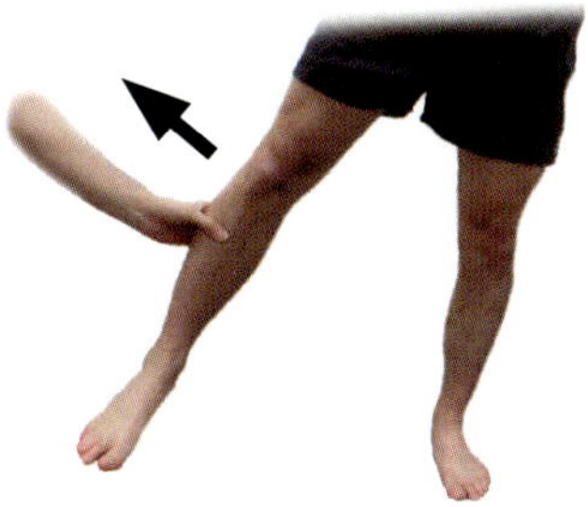

Fig 8.28 The hip abduction test for the gluteal nerve.

Therefore, to broadly test the gluteal nerves, ask the patient to abduct their thigh against resistance, while sitting on the end of the bed. You should apply resistance and palpate the gluteal region.

To request this test from the patient ask them to:
"Keeping your knees straight, can you try to push your thighs out against resistance?"

It is also good practice to test hip extension with the patient lying down to assess the inferior gluteal nerve that innervates the gluteus maximus, although, for the level of the OSPEs, this is not fundamental in practice.

Femoral nerve[84]

The femoral nerve arises from nerve roots L2, L3, and L4, and it travels lateral to the psoas major to enter the femoral triangle. It then divides into superficial and deep branches to provide motor innervation to the quadricep muscles and sensory innervation to the anteromedial thigh, while giving rise to the saphenous nerve branch which provides sensation to the medial side of the leg and the medial side of the foot.

Therefore, to test the femoral nerve, ask the patient to sit on the end of the bed and to extend their knee against resistance. You can also ask the patient to lie supine on the bed and to flex their thigh as a further test, but is not required for the OSPE.

To request this test from the patient ask them to:
"Can you straighten your leg out against resistance?"

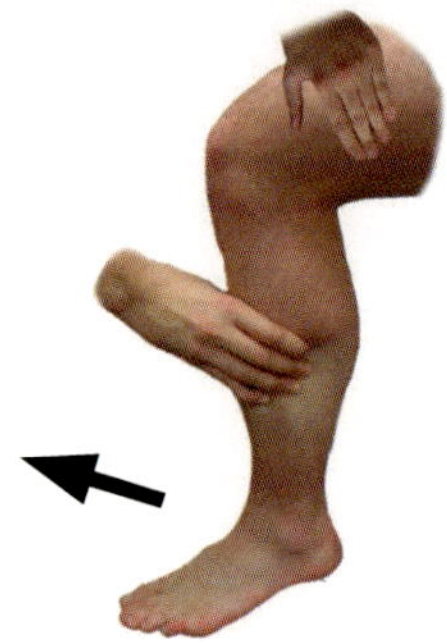

Fig 8.29 The leg extension test for the femoral nerve.

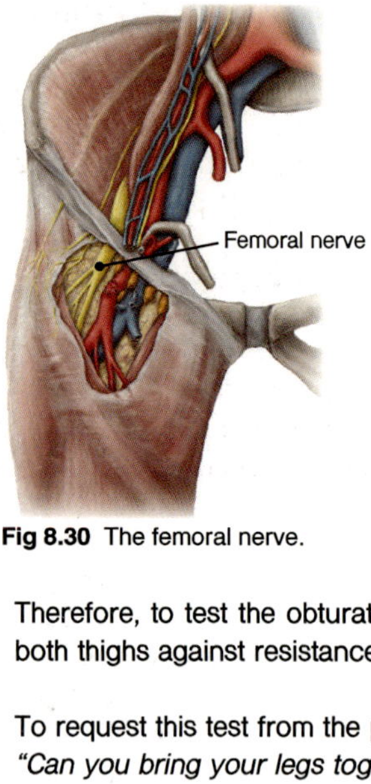

Fig 8.30 The femoral nerve.

Obturator nerve

The obturator nerve arises from the L2, L3, and L4 spinal nerve roots and enters the thigh through the obturator canal (found at the obturator foramen of the pelvis) and divides into an anterior and a posterior branch. The anterior branch then innervates the adductor longus, adductor brevis, and the gracilis muscles whilst giving off a cutaneous branch to provide sensory innervation to a relatively small area on the medial thigh, as highlighted in **Fig 8.32**.

The posterior branch innervates the adductor magnus and the obturator externus (which laterally rotates the thigh at the hip joint).

Therefore, to test the obturator nerve, ask the patient to sit on the end of the bed and to adduct both thighs against resistance.

To request this test from the patient ask them to:
"Can you bring your legs together against resistance?"

Superficial peroneal nerve

The superficial and deep peroneal nerves (originating from L4, L5, and S1 spinal nerve roots) arise from the common fibular nerve (which is one of the main terminal branches of the sciatic nerve). The common fibular nerve descends obliquely along the lateral side of the popliteal fossa to the neck of the fibula, where it then divides.

The superficial peroneal nerve then descends down the fibula to provide motor innervation to the fibularis longus and the fibularis brevis (which function to evert the foot). This one of the reasons (alongside common confusion with the perineal nerve) that the peroneal nerves are commonly referred to as the superficial and deep fibular nerves.

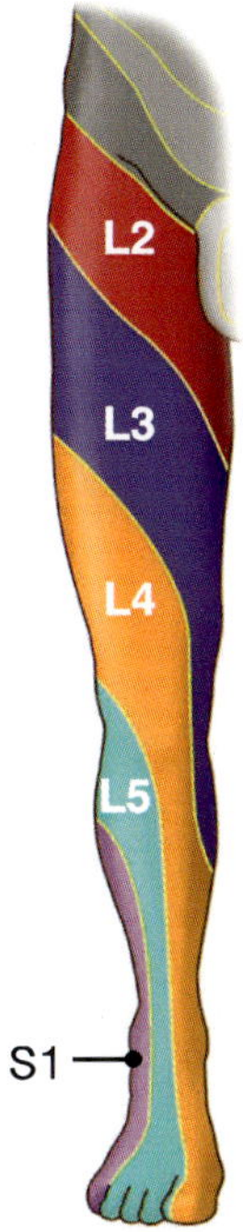

Fig 8.31 The dermatomes of the lower limb

Superficial peroneal nerve

The superficial nerve also provides sensory innervation to anterolateral leg and the dorsum of the foot (except in the space between the hallux and the 2nd digit).

Therefore, to test the superficial peroneal nerve, ask the patient to evert their foot against resistance.

To request this test from the patient ask them to:
"*Can you turn your ankle so that the soles of your feet are facing towards you?*"

Deep peroneal nerve

The deep peroneal nerve is the other terminal branch of common fibular nerve and it descends down the leg more medially to the superficial peroneal nerve, innervating the fibularis tertius (which is a muscle of the anterior compartment of the leg which we did not discuss previously), extensor digitorum longus, extensor hallucis longus, and the tibialis anterior – which all work in the dorsiflexion of the foot. It also provides sensory innervation to a relatively small region on the dorsum of the foot, between the hallux and the 2nd digit, as highlighted in **Fig 8.32**.

Fig 8.32 The peripheral nerve sensation distribution.

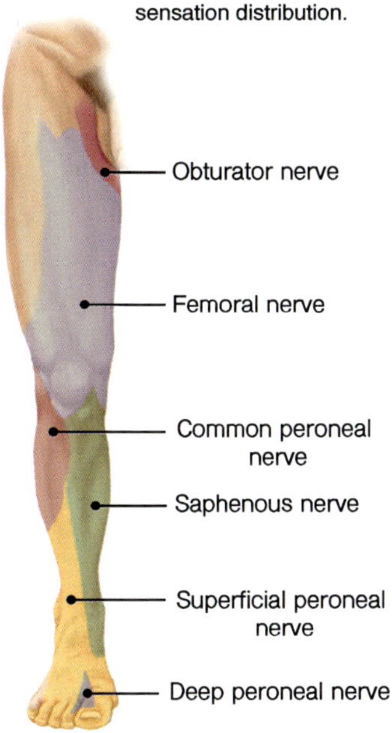

To test the function of this nerve, ask the patient to dorsiflex their foot against resistance by stabilising the ankle joint and placing your hand on the dorsum of the foot. As the extensor digitorum hallucis is also involved, it is also good practice to request hallux dorsiflexion against resistance (stabilise the metatarsophalangeal joint of the hallux).

Sensation of the lower limb

Remember, much like in the upper limb, sensation in the lower limb is categorised into peripheral nerve distribution (which directly assesses sensation of a specific nerve that originates from multiple spinal nerve roots) and dermatomal sensation (which assess sensation from a single spinal nerve root).

In a clinical setting, one assesses the neurological integrity of skin sensation using light touch, pin-prick, proprioception, and vibration.

However, within the OSPE, simple **light-touch sensation** (and perhaps pin-prick sensation at a push) are expected to be the only modalities tested.

Light-touch sensation

Using the wisp of the cotton wool, touch the patient's sternum to establish a central baseline sensation and ask them to confirm once they can feel it.

Then ask the patient close their eyes and to say 'yes' once they feel the wisp of cotton wool touch the skin on their upper limb. It is recommended to begin testing from the C5 dermatome, and to work around the upper limb until the T2 dermatome.

Also assess the contralateral dermatome on the other side of the body before continuing on that limb, and ask the patient whether the sensation felt was the same on both sides.

The comparison of corresponding dermatomes and peripheral nerves on both sides is essential in upper limb sensation testing.

Pin-prick sensation testing, which assesses the spinothalamic tracts, is conducted using the same method as described for light touch sensation, only a neurotip is used in the place of cotton wool.

However, for the individual testing of the cutaneous nerves, please refer to **Fig 8.32** for guidance on anatomical locations.

Reflexes

The two reflexes of interest in the lower limb OSPE are the patellar tendon and the Achilles tendon reflex, both of which are stretch reflexes.

The stretch reflex is the rapid physiological response by a muscle designed as a protective measure against over-stretch. To prevent tearing, the muscle (and the agonistic group of muscles) contracts as a result of an impulse that is sent along the reflex arc, which is not cortically controlled, to the spinal cord and back. This also leads to an inhibition of the antagonistic muscles, which leads to their relaxation.

Therefore, we can use reflex testing to assess nerve function by eliciting a response through the stretch of a muscle tendon which replicates forces capable of tearing the muscle in a non-clinical setting. A stronger than appropriate response/contraction from the muscle as a result of tendon stretch, known as a brisk reflex, is indicative of an upper motor neurone lesion. An absent or weaker than appropriate response/contraction, known as a diminished reflex, is indicative of a lower motor neurone lesion.

Fig 8.33 Striking the tendon hammer on the patellar tendon.

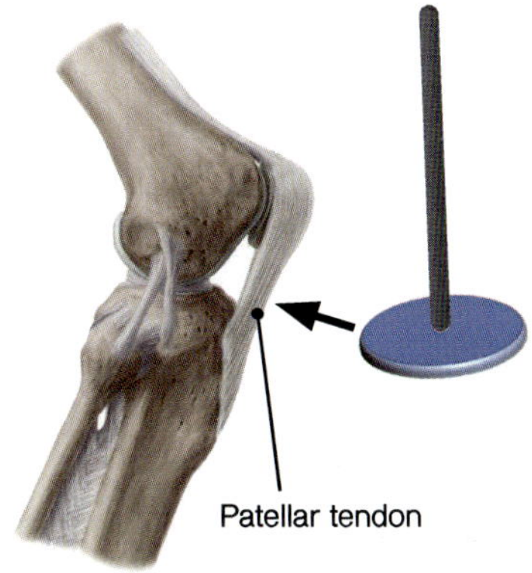

Biceps tendon reflex

You, as the reflex examiner, should strike the tendon directly with your tendon hammer in a motion where the head of the tendon hammer is below the handle.

Although it's certainly possible to elicit a reflex by directing the hammer upwards, the motion of the tendon hammer being pointed downwards much better reflects that of a pendulum and uses gravity to appropriately strike the patellar tendon. Also, it's makes you look much slicker in the OSPE.

If you are having trouble identifying the exact location of the tendon (e.g. if there is a lot of subcutaneous infrapatellar fat - see **Fig 8.6**), place your index finger or your thumb firmly on top of it. Strike your finger, which should then transmit the impulse.
The elicited reflex will cause a slight contraction of the quadriceps, extending the leg.

Although it is not advisable, the test can also be performed with the patient lying down and their entire lower limb supported on your arm. Please note that this something which you should not do in the OSPE, and it is only really used in instances where the patient cannot sit on the end of the bed.

Fig 8.34 Eliciting the patellar tendon reflex.

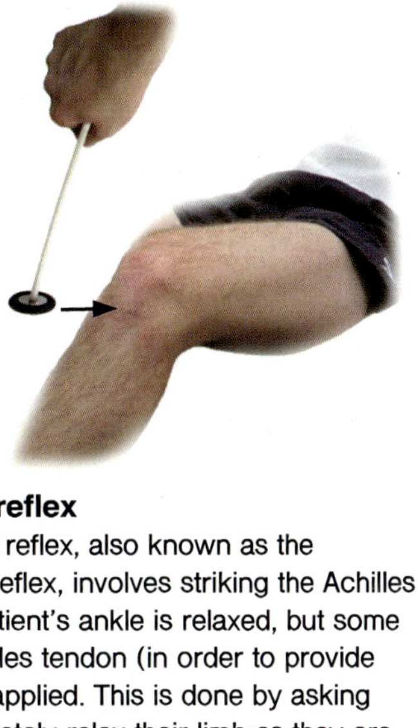

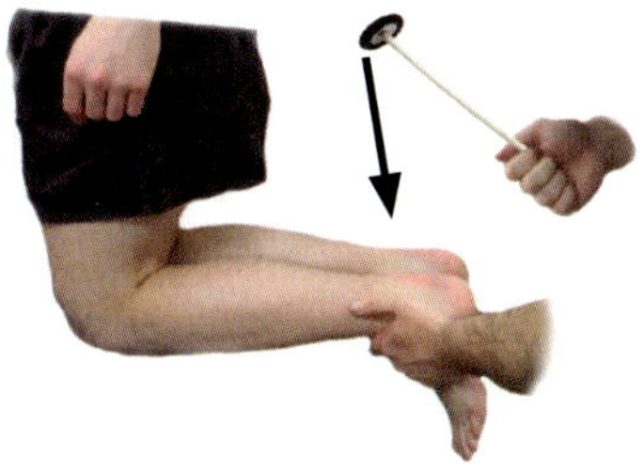

Fig 8.35 Eliciting the calcaneal tendon reflex.

Achilles tendon reflex

The Achilles tendon reflex, also known as the calcaneal or ankle reflex, involves striking the Achilles tendon while the patient's ankle is relaxed, but some tension on the Achilles tendon (in order to provide efficient stretch) is applied. This is done by asking the patient to completely relax their limb as they are lying on the bed, whilst you, as the examiner, hold the patient's foot and initiate dorsiflexion to an extent. Do you not overdo the dorsiflexion of the foot as the ankle jerk will not work.

This procedure can also be performed with the patient sitting on their knees on the end of the bed, with their feet hanging of the bed the soles facing the examiner.

Jendrassik manoeuvre

If no response has been observed after two attempts of trying to elicit a reflex in the lower limb, consider the use of the Jendrassik manoeuvre. This is a manoeuvre where the patient clenches their teeth and interlocks both sets of flexed fingers into a hook-like form. Its mechanism is still not yet completely clear, but it often leads to a larger response when doing a lower limb reflex test as it has been suggested to prevent the conscious inhibitory mechanism resisting this response.[85]

4 The arterial supply of the lower limb

Once the external iliac artery (terminal branch of the aorta) crosses under the inguinal ligament, it becomes the femoral artery. This artery is the main artery of the lower limb and it passes through the femoral triangle where it gives off five branches and continues to descend down posterolaterally to form the popliteal artery.

Extra medical knowledge

The femoral pulse can be felt using the tips of your 2nd, 3rd, and 4th digits midway between the ASIS and the pubic symphyses. If there is a lot of subcutaneous fat, you will need to push firmly. You will not be asked to palpate the femoral artery in the OSPE.

The popliteal artery then descends down in the posterior compartment of the thigh, and shortly after crossing the popliteal fossa, it gives rise to the anterior and posterior tibial arteries.

The popliteal pulse can be found at the midline in the inferior part popliteal fossa of the patient while their knee is flexed to relax the hamstring.

The posterior tibial artery then gives rise to the fibular artery while it continues inferiorly. Together, these three arteries supply blood to the leg. The posterior tibial artery also supplies blood to the plantar side of the foot, while partly supplying the digits also.

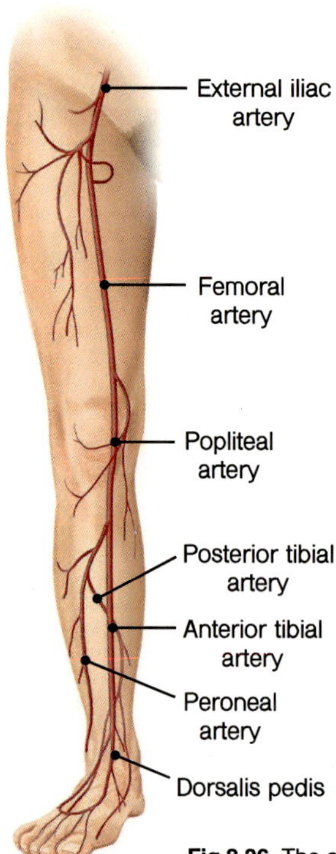

Fig 8.36 The arteries of the lower limb.

The posterior tibial artery pulse can be palpated behind and below the medial malleolus, by holding the ankle of the patient while they are lying on the bed.

The dorsalis pedis, which is a continuation of the anterior tibial artery, supplies the dorsal side of the foot.

The dorsalis pedis pulse is palpable on the dorsum of the foot in the first intermetatarsal space just lateral to the extensor digitorum hallucis tendon.

5 The venous drainage of the lower limb

Much like the veins of the upper limb, the venous system of the lower limb can be divided into the superficial and deep veins.

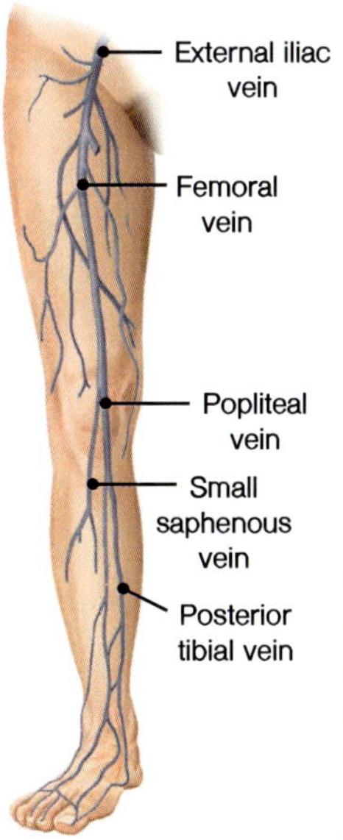

Fig 8.37 The veins of the lower limb.

The deep veins, again, much like the upper limb, accompany the arteries down the lower limb. For the purposes of the OSPE, knowledge of the deep veins of the leg can be minimal, and the superficial veins are of more importance for the lower limb station.

The superficial veins are found in the subcutaneous and they drain into the deep veins of the lower limb. There are two superficial veins that are of significant importance for the OSPE; the great saphenous vein and the small saphenous vein.

The long saphenous vein is formed by the dorsal venous arch of the foot and the dorsal vein of the hallux, and it drains into the femoral vein at the femoral triangle, immediately inferior to the inguinal ligament that makes up the base of the triangle
The vein ascends up the medial side of the lower limb, passing anteriorly to the medial malleolus at the ankle, which is a relatively easy area to locate the vein.

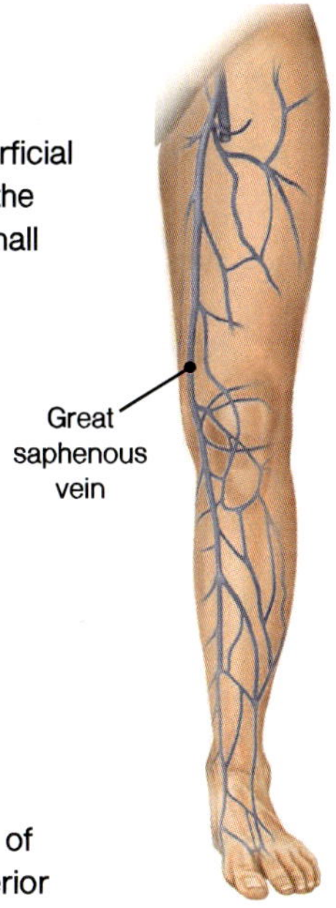

Fig 8.38 The great saphenous vein.

The small saphenous vein is also formed by the dorsal venous arch of the foot, and the dorsal vein of the fifth digit. It ascends on the posterior side of the leg, passing posteriorly to the lateral malleolus and along the lateral border of the calcaneal tendon. It then drains into the popliteal vein in the popliteal fossa, between the two heads of the gastrocnemius muscle.

Extra medical knowledge

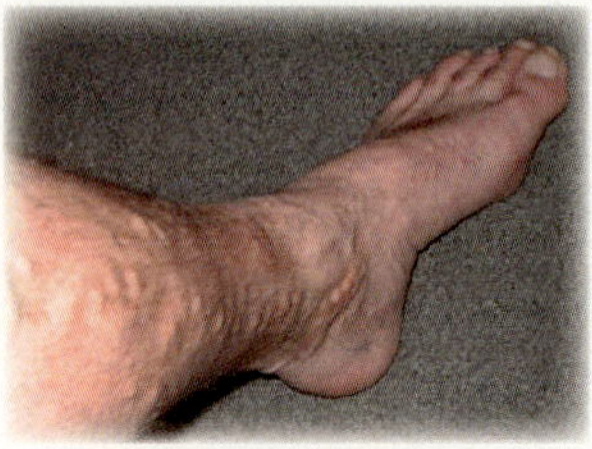

Fig 8.39 Varicose veins.

Varicose veins is a condition associated with the incompetency of the valves of the superficial veins, which exist to prevent the backflow of blood from the deep veins.[86] When these valves become incompetent and the blood flows back into these superficial veins, the increased intra-luminal pressure causes the veins to dilates and become tortuous – varicose veins. This condition can be very painful if chronic, and it can cause brown discolouration of the distal leg.[86]

6 Borders and contents of the relevant lower limb structures

Guteal safe area

When administering certain intramuscular medications, the gluteal safe area (also known as the ventrogluteal site) is the site that is used for the injection. This site is located in the superior lateral region of the gluteal space so as to minimise the risk of damage to the sciatic nerve, found in the inferior medial region of the gluteal space. You may be asked to describe, and even demonstrate this gluteal safe area on the patient during the OSPE. Demonstration will require more than just pointing to the superior lateral region, and it is good practice to know the hand positioning required of the practitioner administering the injection.

The heel of the positioning hand must be placed on the greater trochanter of the femur with the fingers pointing superiorly. The second digit (index finger) is then placed on the ASIS, while the lateral three fingers are placed posteriorly on the iliac crest, forming a 'V' shape with the fingers. The injection is then administered in the centre of that 'V'shape created.

Femoral triangle

The femoral triangle is a wedge-shaped depression formed in the medial aspect of the thigh, where many large neurovascular structures pass through.

Its borders are formed by the inguinal ligament (the superior border – or base of the triangle), the sartorius muscle (the lateral border), and the adductor longus muscle (medial border).

It contains, from laterally to medially; the femoral nerve, the femoral artery, the femoral vein, the femoral canal, and the lymphatic vessels (found within the femoral canal).

Fig 8.40 The femoral triangle

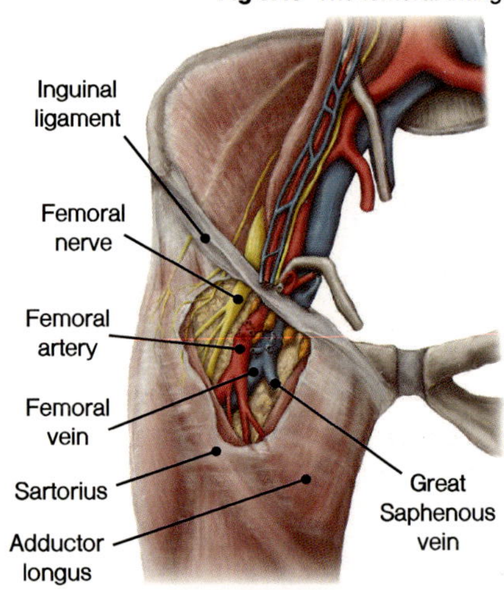

The femoral artery, femoral vein, and the femoral canal are enclosed within a fascia, known as the femoral sheath. The long saphenous vein also drains into the femoral vein within the femoral triangle, and this is important to note. The femoral canal also contains empty space to allow for distension of the femoral vein to cope with an increased venous.

A popular acronym for the contents is: NAVEL; nerve, artery, vein, empty space (of the femoral canal), and lymphatic vessel.
Please don't forget the long saphenous vein also!

The popliteal fossa

The popliteal fossa is a 2.5 cm wide, diamond-shaped depression located posteriorly to the knee joint.

The popliteal fossa is a diamond-shaped depression located posterior to the knee joint. Though it mainly consists of connective tissue, important nerves and vessels traverse this area to enter the leg from the thigh.

The superolateral border of the popliteal fossa is bound biceps femoris, and the superomedial border is bound by the semimembranosus and the semitendinosus muscles.

The inferomedial border is formed by the medial head of the gastrocnemius, and the inferolateral border is formed from the lateral head of the gastrocnemius and plantaris muscle.

Fig 8.41 The popliteal fossa

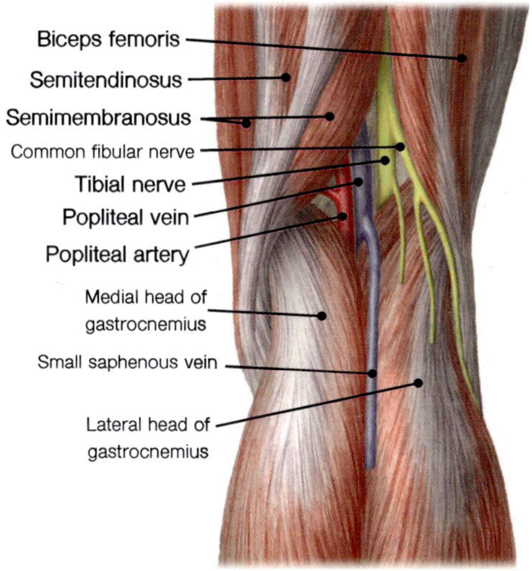

Its contents, from lateral to medial, are: the common fibular nerve, the tibial nerve, the popliteal vein, and the popliteal artery.

The common fibular nerve and the tibular nerve are terminal branches of the sciatic nerve, and lie the most superficial in the popliteal fossa.

The small saphenous vein also enters the popliteal fossa by piercing the popliteal fascia to drain into the popliteal vein, which is a continuation of the posterior tibial vein (one of the deep veins in the leg).

The popliteal artery, which is the continuation of the femoral artery, gives rise to five genicular arteries which supply and anastomose anteriorly to the knee joint.

Medical Imaging

By Arian Arjomandi Rad

Introduction to the chapter

First of all, you need to be able to distinguish between a CT image, MRI image and x-rays. You should also be able to comment on when each modality would be preferred. Moreover, identifying some basic pathologies would definitely be useful.

CT scans are cheaper and quicker than MRI's so are preferred in cases of trauma or when bone pathologies are suspected. MRI's give greater soft tissue detail so are preferred when looking for subtler abnormalities like neurological conditions of brain tissues.
For instance, in the case of HNS, CT scans are more common than MRI scans.

Types of view in imaging is exactly as it's described in anatomical terms. A mid-sagittal view is taken from the midline, and you'll see a nice front to back view of midline structures. It is able to form a good depiction between anterior and posterior structures. An axial slice is through the horizontal plane, and can depict a connection between structures on opposite sides of the body. A coronal view is front to back and can depict the connection between superior and inferior structures well.

The most important aspect for you to learn at this stage is being able to identify the different structures in a radiograph from a healthy patient.

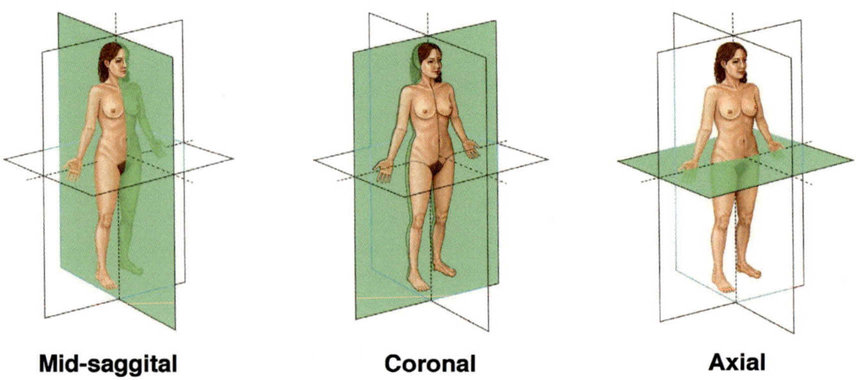

Fig 9.1 Body planes

X-ray

X-ray radiographs are some of the most commonly used types of imaging as they are relatively cheap and easy to obtain. In this type of imaging, a small amount of radiation is passed through the body area of interest, and this is then is captured on a film.
X-ray radiographs are mainly used to assess bone fractures or dislocation, locate foreign objects present in the body, assess for infections (e.g. pneumonia), and to visualise the presence of disease such as tumours/malignancy/deterioration.[87] This type of imaging lets us visualize the internal organs such as the heart, lungs, pulmonary airways, vessels and internal abdominal organs. There are several types of x-rays radiographs which you might encounter based on the modality and projection used. In the case of chest x-rays, they could be posterior-anterior (PA), anterior-posterior (AP), or lateral.
An interesting and useful fact is that PA x-rays are the most commonly used and that you cannot comment on the size of the heart in a AP radiograph.

In x-rays bones will stain white as they absorb most of the radiation, while air spaces will be of black colour.

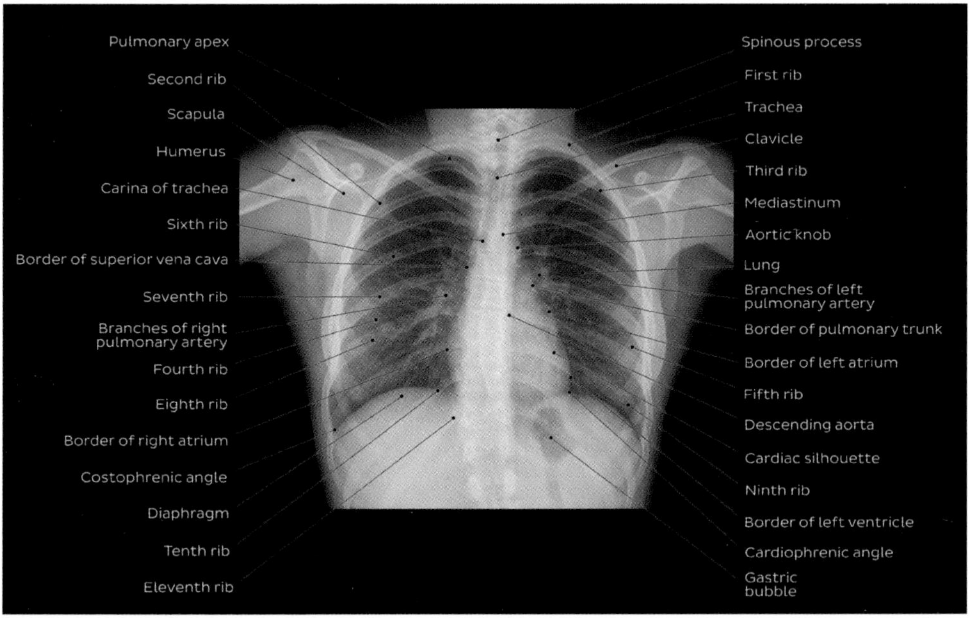

Fig 9.2 PA chest x-ray radiograph illustrating the structures in the heart.

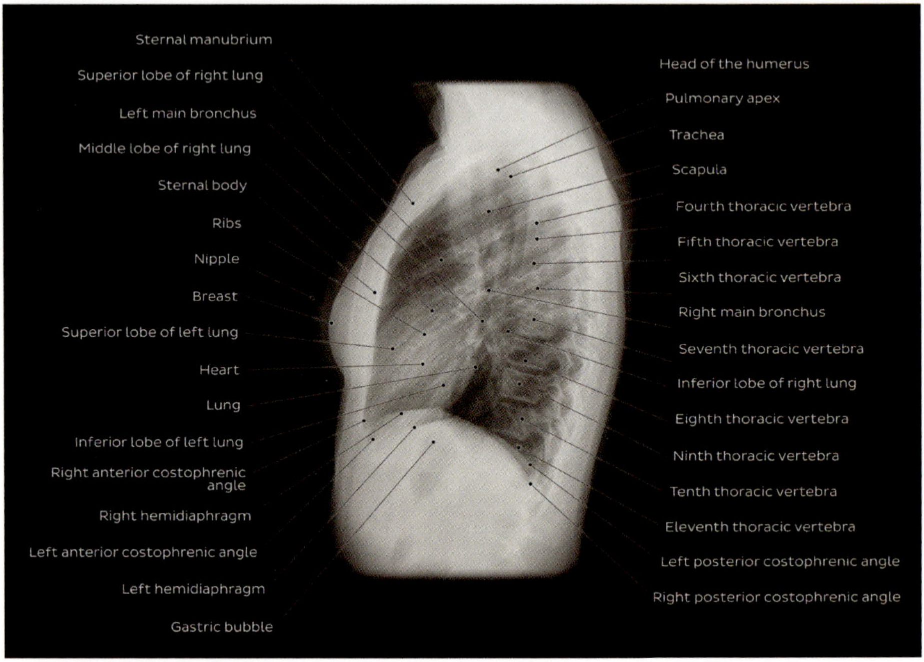

Fig 9.3 Lateral chest x-ray illustrating the structures in the chest.

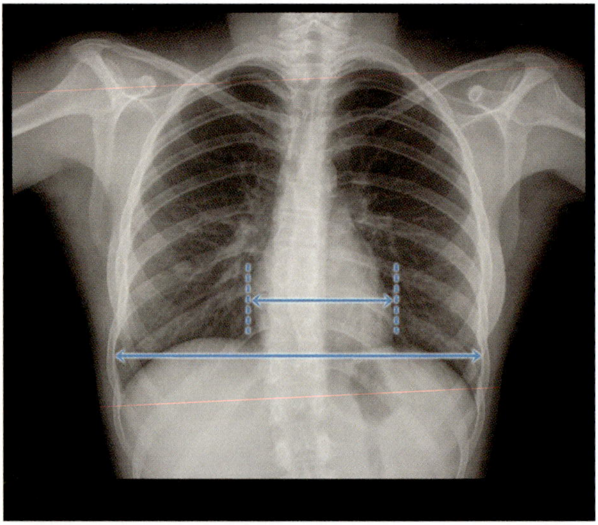

The image on the left illustrates how to calculate the cardiothoracic ratio which is used to assess for any enlargement of the cardiac silhouette, a sign of cardiomegaly.

This is carried out by calculating the ratio of the horizontal cardiac diameter to the horizontal thoracic diameter. This should in a healthy subject be less than 0.5.[87]

Fig 9.4 Chest x-ray image demonstrating how to calculate the CTR value.

Computed tomography (CT) scans

CT scans are a relatively new and popular type of imagining modality which join x-rays and computer processes to obtain 360° image sections of specific anatomical areas within the body. CT images are can be obtained in a short period of time (5-15 minutes)[88], which makes them really efficient and popular in emergency settings where for instance a haemorrhage needs to be spotted in the shortest period possible. The drawback of CT scans is the relatively high amount of radiation to which patients are exposed to and the risk of developing cancer.[88]

CT scans also have a high resolution which allows us to efficiently differentiate between structures within the body. As with X-rays, CT scans also focus on different parts of the body and this includes, but is not limited to, CT Head (one of the most common), CT Chest and CT Abdomen. Some examples of pathologies which may be spotted with a CT scan are liver, pancreas, and kidney masses with CT Abdomen; emphysema, pulmonary embolism, aortic aneurysm, coronary artery disease (CAD), pleural effusions, and lung tumours through CT chest; tumours, haemorrhages or flow obstruction thorough CT Head.[88]

Furthermore, it is important to point out that CT scans might not be appropriate for pregnant woman and children. Instead, MRI or ultrasound scans might be preferred with those patients.

Similarly to x-ray radiographs, on CT scans bones will stain white due to their high absorbance of radiation, while air will show up as black.

Interesting facts about CT head scan - *by Samuel Hammond*

Type of Haemorrhage	How it looks on CT
Extradural	Lens-shaped, hyperdense (white) region [Arterial blood] Does not pass the suture lines – this is where the dura mater attaches to the skull.
Subdural	Crescent-shaped, hyperdense region. Can cross suture lines
Subarachnoid	White/grey areas in the ventricles and cisterns since blood is flowing into the spaces where CSF is usually stored.

CT Head Scan Pathologies: [88,89]

The structures to identify in the OSPE for imaging will be the gross, overall structures, such as the parietal bone, since smaller structures take a good level of skill to visualise. The best way to learn structures on imaging modalities is to look at scans without labels, try to identify as many structures as possible, and check if you're correct.

In terms of other pathologies – stroke imaging on CT scans is very common. The difference between haemorrhagic and ischaemic is very important in terms of the management – since ischaemic strokes tend to be caused by a clot of some form (blocking blood flow), the treatment is clot busters and anti-coagulants, which would be catastrophic in patients with haemorrhagic strokes. So, knowing how to distinguish between them is literally the difference between life and death.

As I mentioned previously, hyperdense white areas show bleeding and indicate active bleeds/fresh blood – so will be present on a haemorrhagic stroke scan.

In ischaemic stroke, you won't see much on an early CT scan. It's proper practice to take more CT scans 4+ hours after the stroke presentation – you'll start to see dark patches where tissue is dying due to ischaemia.

Imaging is tough and there's a reason medicine relies on specialist radiologists to look over the scans. My advice is to use a combination of diagrams and scans to learn the anatomy of the head, neck and spine to ensure you're an expert in anatomical and radiological means.

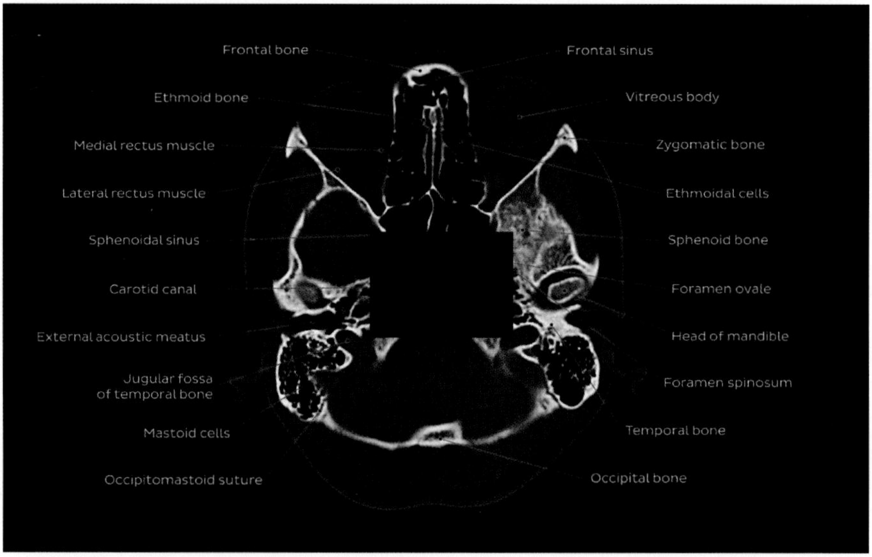

Fig 9.5 Axial CT scan at the level of the jugular fossa

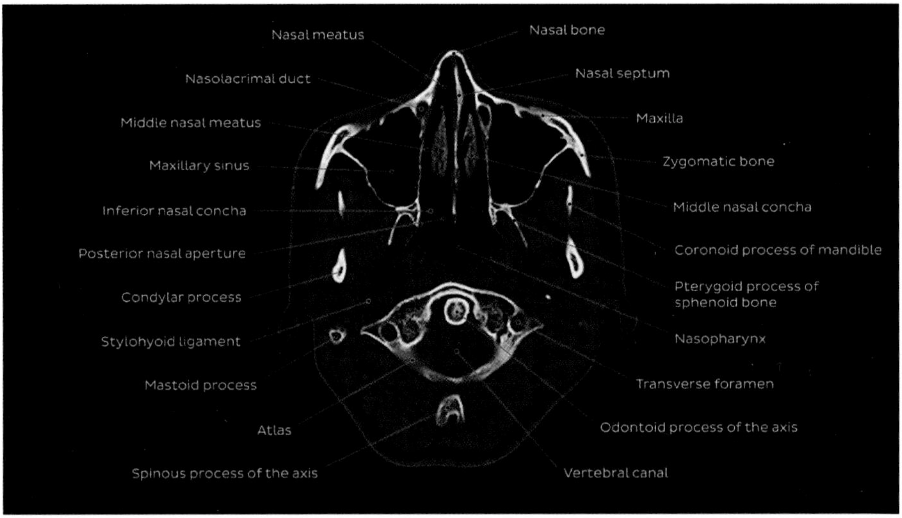

Fig 9.6 Axial CT scan at the level of the first cervical vertebra

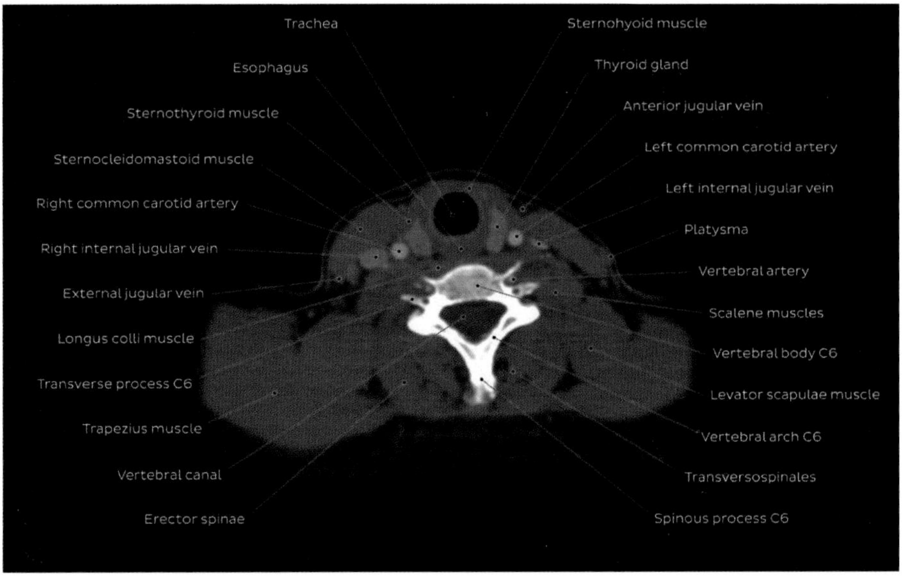

Fig 9.7 Axial CT at the level of the sixth cervical vertebra

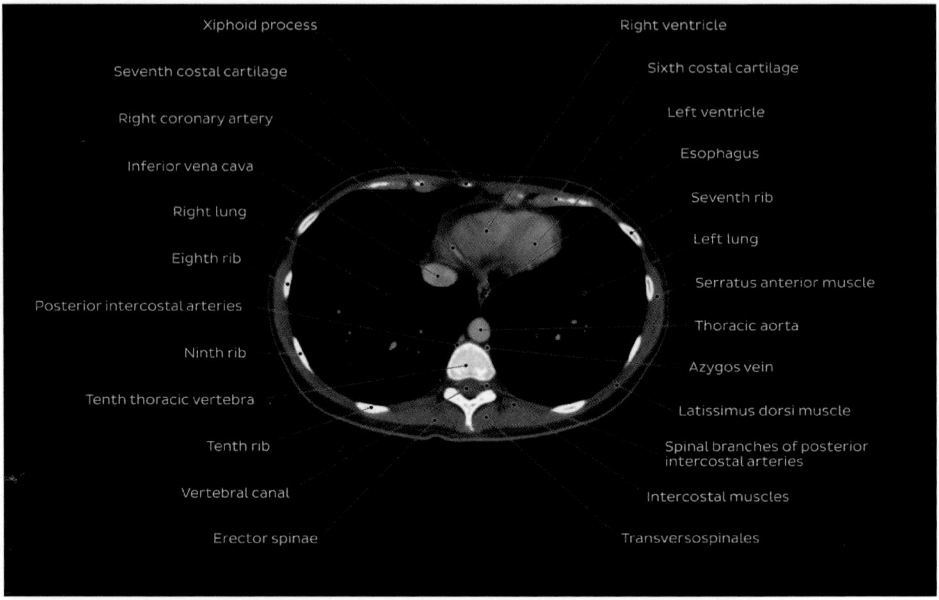

Fig 9.8 T10 level thoracic axial CT scan

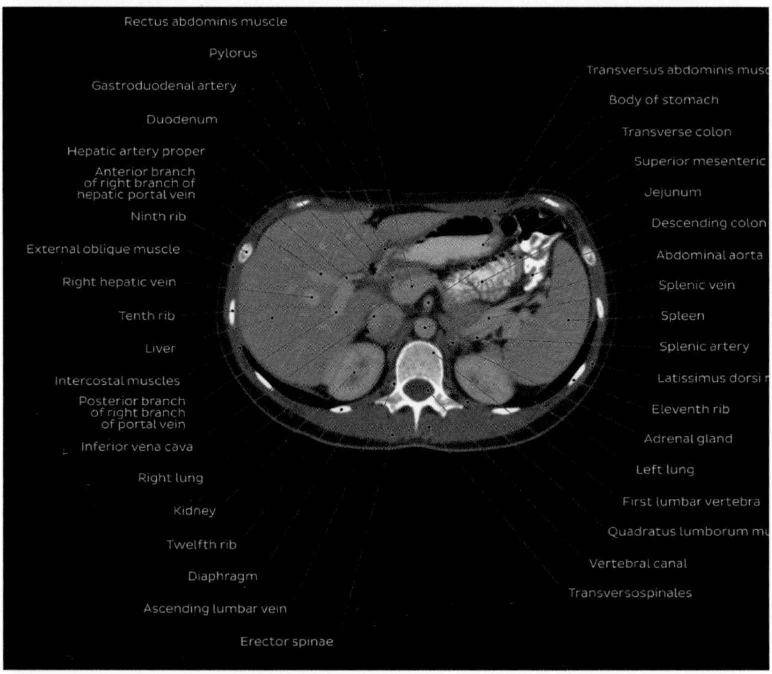

Fig 9.9 L1 level axial CT Abdomen

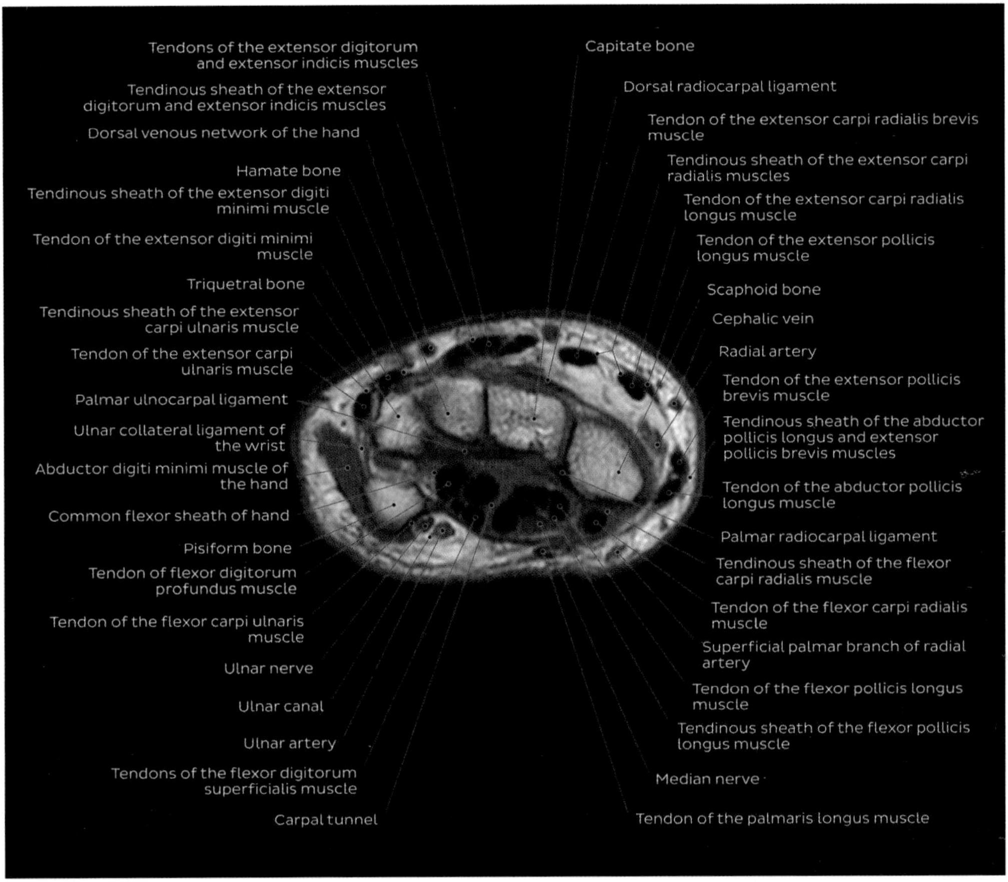

Fig 9.10 Axial CT scan of the Carpal Tunnel

Magnetic Resonance Imaging (MRI)

Unlike the other two types of imaging, MRI does not make use of ionizing radiation but it makes use of magnetic fields and radio waves to create high quality images. The use of these magnetics fields makes MRI scans capable of very precisely differentiating between tissues. Consequently, in several pathologies involving soft tissues, MRI scans tend to be preferred over CT scans. On the other hand, MRI scans take longer time (even up to hours for some parts of the body) making them inconvenient when compared to CT scans, especially in emergency settings.[90]

Moreover, when staging cancers MRI scans tend to be the method of choice. Some examples in which MRI scans are usually used to aid the diagnosis included Epilepsy, Myocardial Ischemia, Myocarditis, Congenital Heart Disease, Aneurysm, lesions of abdominal organs such as liver, pancreas and bile ducts and demyelinating diseases (e.g. Multiple Sclerosis).[91]

There are different types of sequences which could be used in MRI scans, thus providing different colours based on the sequence used. The imaging characteristics are more complicated than the previous CT scan, the tissues have different brightness. Usually air and bone both appear black while fat and soft tissues appear bright.

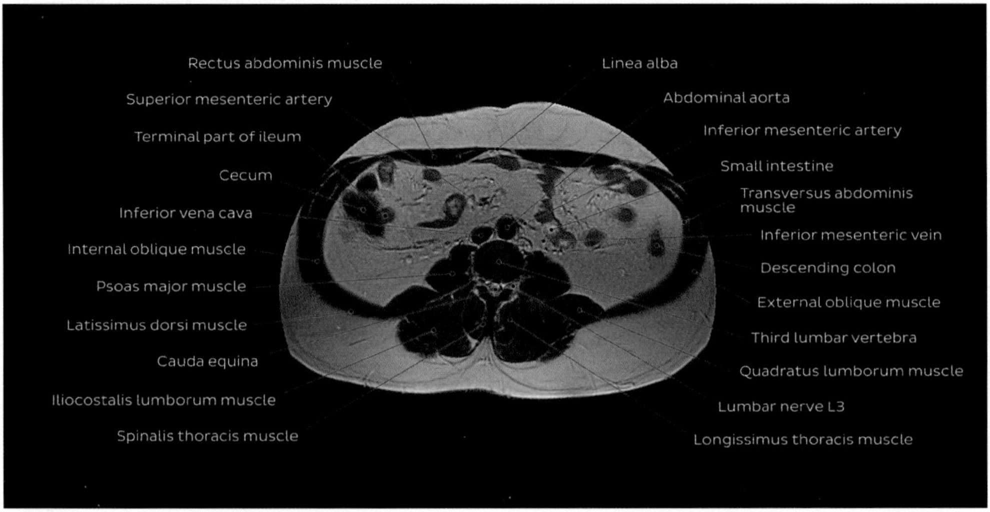

Fig 9.11 Abdominal MRI 3rd lumbar level

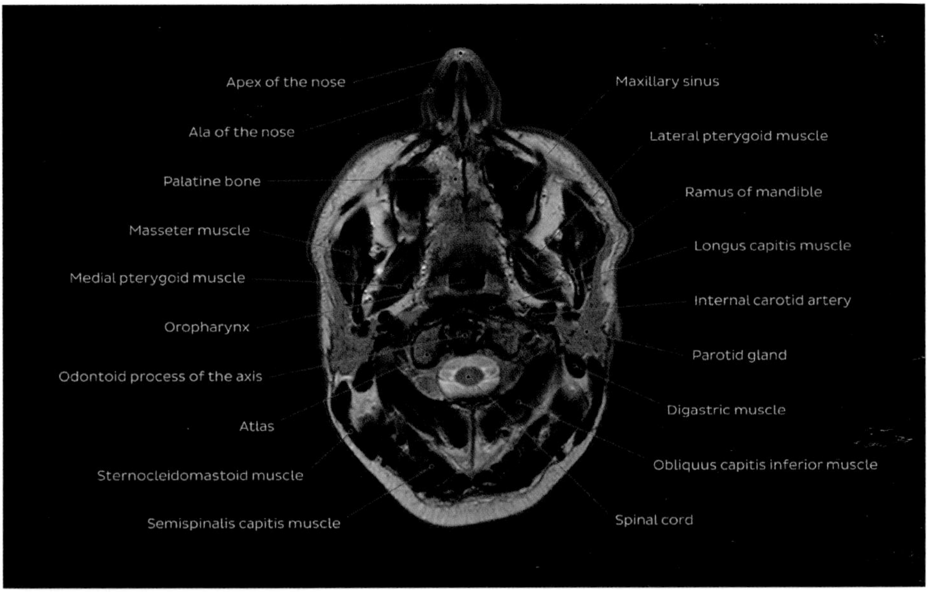

Fig 9.12 MRI axial first cervical level

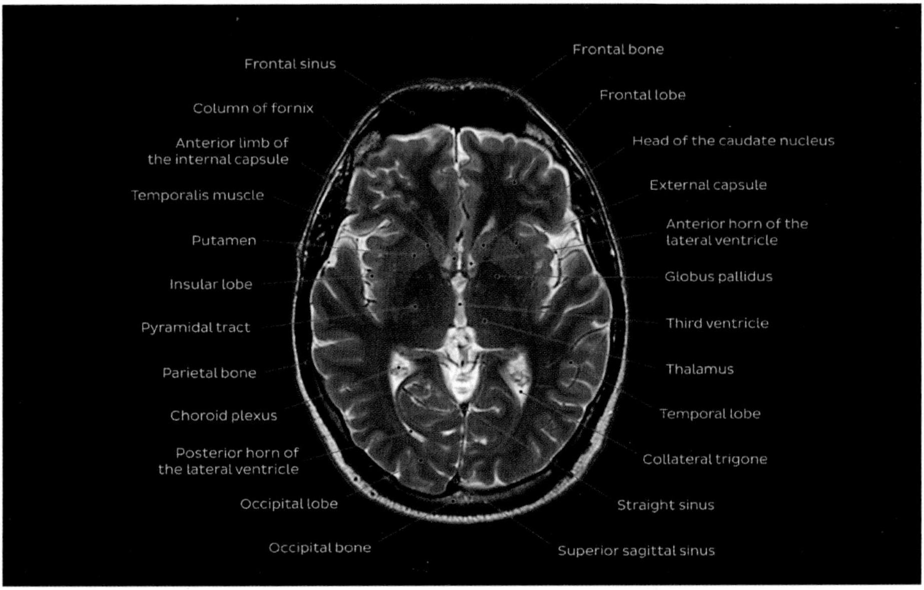

Fig 9.13 Axial MRI caudate nucleus level

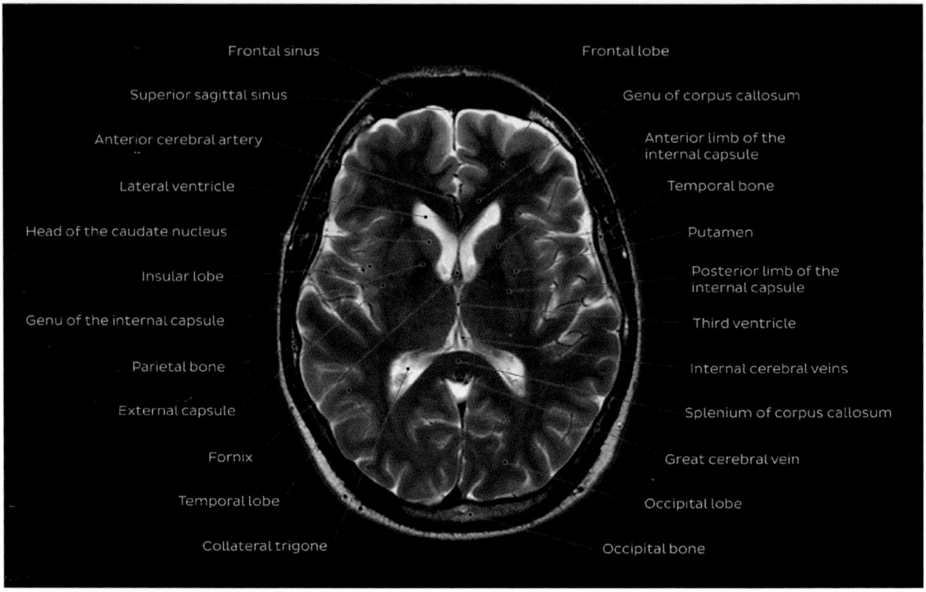

Fig 9.14 Axial MRI thalamus level

References

1. Perkins GD, Lockey AS, Belder MAD, Moore F, Weissberg P, Gray H. National initiatives to improve outcomes from out-of-hospital cardiac arrest in England. *Emergency Medicine Journal.* 2015;33(7): 448–451.
2. Weisfeldt ML, Everson-Stewart S, Sitlani C, Rea T, Aufderheide TP, Atkins DL, et al. Ventricular Tachyarrhythmias after Cardiac Arrest in Public versus at Home. *New England Journal of Medicine.* 2011;364(4): 313–321.
3. Govender C, Colquhoun M, Deakin C, Handley A, Smith C, Smyth M. Adult basic life support and automated external defibrillation. *Resuscitation Council (UK) Guidelines 2015.* Resuscitation Council (UK)
4. Perkins GD, Handley AJ, Koster KW, et al. European Resuscitation Council Guidelines for Resuscitation 2015 Section 2 Adult basic life support and automated external defibrillation. *Resuscitation* 2015:95:81-98.
5. Larsen MP, Eisenberg MS, Cummins RO, Hallstrom AP. Predicting survival from out-of-hospital cardiac arrest: A graphic model. *Annals of Emergency Medicine.* 1993;22(11): 1652–1658.
6. Hasselqvist-Ax I, Riva G, Herlitz J, Rosenqvist M, Hollenberg J, Nordberg P, et al. Early Cardiopulmonary Resuscitation in Out-of-Hospital Cardiac Arrest. *New England Journal of Medicine.* 2015;372(24): 2307–2315.
7. Valenzuela TD, Roe DJ, Nichol G, Clark LL, Spaite DW, Hardman RG. Outcomes of Rapid Defibrillation by Security Officers After Cardiac Arrest in Casinos. *New England Journal Medicine.* 2000;343:1206–9.
8. Association AHA. Basic Life Support (BLS) Provider Manual. 1st ed. *American Heart Association*; 2016.
9. Cheskes S, Schmicker RH, Verbeek PR, Salcido DD, Brown SP, Brooks S, et al. The impact of shock pause on survival from out-of-hospital shockable cardiac arrest during the Resuscitation Outcomes Consortium PRIMED trial. *Resuscitation.* 2014;85(3): 336–342.
10. Stiell IG, Brown SP, Christenson J, Cheskes S, Nichol G, Powell J, et al. What is the role of chest compression depth during out-of-hospital cardiac arrest resuscitation?. *Critical Care Medicine.* 2012;40(4): 1192–1198.
11. Stiell IG, Brown SP, Nichol G, Cheskes S, Vaillancourt C, Callaway CW, et al. What Is the Optimal Chest Compression Depth During Out-of-Hospital Cardiac Arrest Resuscitation of Adult Patients? *Circulation.* 2014;130(22): 1962–1970.
12. Aufderheide TP, Pirrallo RG, Yannopoulos D, Klein JP, Briesen CV, Sparks CW, et al. Incomplete chest wall decompression: A clinical evaluation of CPR performance by trained laypersons and an assessment of alternative manual chest compression–decompression techniques. *Resuscitation.* 2006;71(3): 341–351.
13. Heimlich HJ, Patrick EA. The Heimlich maneuver. *Postgraduate Medicine.* 1990;87(6): 38–53.
14. Guildner CW, Williams D, Subitch T. Airway obstructed by foreign material: The Heimlich maneuver. *Journal of the American College of Emergency Physicians.* 1976;5(9): 675–677.
15. Drake R, Vogl W, Mitchell A. *Gray's Anatomy for Students.* 3rd Ed. Elsevier. 2014.
16. Smith L, Brown J, Quint J. *Respiratory Medicine.* JP Medical Publishers. 2015.
17. Walker HK et al. *Clinical Methods: The History, Physical, and Laboratory Examinations.* 3rd Ed. Boston: Butterworths. 1990.
18. Sarkar M et al. Auscultation of the respiratory system. *Annals of Thoracic Medicine.* 2015;10(3):158.
19. Meenakshi S, Manjunath K.Y, Balasubramanyam V. Morphological variations of the lung fissures and lobes. *Indian J. Chest Dis Allied Sci* 2004;46:179-182.
20. Laws D. BTS guidelines for the insertion of a chest drain. *Thorax.* 2003;58(90002): 53ii–59. 21.
21. British Heart Foundation: Cardiovascular Disease Fact Sheet . *British Heart Foundation*; 2018.
22. Florin MF. *Atlas of Heart Anatomy and Development.* Springer London Ltd; 2016.

23. Innes JA, Dover AR, Fairhurst K. *Macleods clinical examination.* Edinburgh: Elsevier; 2018.

24. Rajaganeshan R, Ludlam CL, Francis DP, Parasramka SV, Sutton R. Accuracy in ECG lead placement among technicians, nurses, general physicians and cardiologists. *International Journal of Clinical Practice.* 2007;62(1): 65–70.

25. Dock W. Mode Of Production Of The First Heart Sound. *Archives of Internal Medicine.* 1933;51(5): 737.

26. Stein PD, Sabbah H. Second Heart Sound. *American Journal of Noninvasive Cardiology.* 1987;1(1): 68–72.

27. Sabbah HN, Stein PD. Turbulent blood flow in humans: its primary role in the production of ejection murmurs. *Circulation Research.* 1976;38(6): 513–525.

28. Collins SP, Lindsell CJ, Peacock WF, Hedger VD, Askew J, Eckert DC, et al. The Combined Utility of an S3 Heart Sound and B-Type Natriuretic Peptide Levels in Emergency Department Patients With Dyspnea. *Journal of Cardiac Failure.* 2006;12(4): 286–292.

29. Rectra EH. Audibility of the Fourth Heart Sound. *JAMA.* 1972;221(1): 36.

30. Braunwald E, Aygen MM. Idiopathic myocardial hypertrophy without congestive heart failure or obstruction to blood flow. *The American Journal of Medicine.* 1963;35(1): 7–19.

31. McGee SR. *Evidence-based physical diagnosis.* 3rd ed. Philadelphia: Saunders; 2012.

32. Hall JE. *Guyton and Hall textbook of medical physiology.* 13th ed. Saunders; 2016.

33. Standring S, Ananad N, Gray H. *Grays anatomy the anatomical basis of clinical practice*; 41st ed. Philadelphia, PA: Elsevier; 2016.

34. Anderson RH, Razavi R, Taylor AM. Cardiac anatomy revisited. *Journal of Anatomy.* 2004;205(3): 159–177.

35. Smith GT. The anatomy of the coronary circulation. *The American Journal of Cardiology.* 1962;9(3): 327–342.

36. Moore K, Dalley A, Agur A. *Clinical Oriented Anatomy.* 6th ed. United States of America: Lippincott Williams & Wilkins.; 2010.

37. Abbas AK, Aster JC, Kumar V. *Robbins and Cotran Pathologic basis of disease.* 9th ed. Saunders; 2015.

38. Goodman S. *Anatomy: The Abdomen.* Available from: https://www.kumc.edu/AMA-MSS/Study/abdomen.htm. [Accessed on 21st November 2018]

39. Naylor CD. Physical Examination of the Liver. *JAMA.* 1994;271(23):1859–1865.

40. Ahmed F, Fogel E. Right Upper Quadrant Pain and a Normal Abdominal Ultrasound. *Clinical Gastroenterology and Hepatology.* 2008; 6 (11): 1198-1201.

41. Katritsis E, Papadopoulos N. First Chapter: Digestive System. *Anatomy of the Human.* Greece: Medical Publications Litsa; 2016. pp. 11-114.

42. Lerma EV. Approach to the Patient with Renal Disease. *Primary Care: Clinics in Office Practice.* 2008;35(2): 183–194.

43. Faiz O, Blackburn S, Moffat D. *Anatomy at a Glance.* Hoboken: John Wiley & Sons, Incorporated; 2011.

44. Fehrenbach MJ, Herring SW. *Illustrated anatomy of the head and neck.* 5th ed. St. Louis, MO: Elsevier; 2017.

45. Odell EW. *Clinical problem solving in dentistry.* 3rd ed. Edinburgh: Churchill Livingstone, Elsevier; 2014.

46. Tortora GJ, Derrickson B. *Principles of anatomy and physiology.* 3rd ed. Hoboken, NJ: Wiley; 2009.

47. Erman A, Kejner A, Hogikyan N, Feldman E. Disorders of Cranial Nerves IX and X. *Seminars in Neurology.* 2009;29(01): 085–092.

48. Yanoff M, Duker JS. *Ophthalmology.* 3rd ed. Edinburgh: Mosby; 2008.

49. Fincham EF. The Accommodation Reflex and its Stimulus. *British Journal of Ophthalmology.* 1951;35(7): 381–393.

50. Adler FH, Levin LA, Kaufman PL, Alm A. *Adlers physiology of the eye.* 11th ed. Edinburgh: Saunders Elsevier; 2011.

51. Lee IH, Miller NR, Zan E, Tavares F, Blitz AM, Sung H, et al. Visual Defects in Patients With Pituitary Adenomas: The Myth of Bitemporal Hemianopsia. *American Journal of Roentgenology.* 2015;205(5)

52. Ellis H. Applied anatomy of cricothyrotomy and tracheostomy. *British Journal of Hospital Medicine.* 2009;70(Sup10).

53. Cole LK. Otoscopic evaluation of the ear canal. *Veterinary Clinics of North America: Small Animal Practice.* 2004;34(2): 397–410.

54. Bannon M, Heller S, Rivera M. Anatomic considerations for central venous cannulation. *Risk Management and Healthcare Policy.* 2011; 27.

55. Mulroy MF, Norris MC, Liu SS. Safety Steps for Epidural Injection of Local Anesthetics. *Survey of Anesthesiology.* 1998;42(6): 352.

56. Magee D, Sueki D. *Orthopedic Physical Assessment Atlas.* 6th ed. London: Elsevier Health Sciences; 2013.

57. Yi JW, Kim DH, Heo YM, Jun JB. Bilateral sternoclavicular joint dislocation due to sternal fracture: Is it a dislocation or a separation? *Archives of Orthopaedic and Trauma Surgery.* 2016;136(5): 605–608.

58. Krøner K, Lind T, Jensen J. The epidemiology of shoulder dislocations. *Archives of Orthopaedic and Trauma Surgery.* 1989;108(5): 288–290.

59. Almaiyah M, Handoll H, Rangan A. Surgical versus non-surgical treatment for acute anterior shoulder dislocation. *The Cochrane Database of Systematic Reviews.* 2003

60. Bhatt C, Prajapati B, Patil D, Patel V, Singh G, Mehta C. Variation in the insertion of the latissimus dorsi & its clinical importance. *Journal of Orthopaedics.* 2013;10(1):25-28.

61. Saladin KS. *Anatomy & physiology: the unity of form and function.* 7th ed. New York: McGraw-Hill; 2015.

62. Chia J. Anatomy Of The Upper Limb. *The Scientific Basis of Tissue Transplantation.* 2001; 3–24.

63. Sebastin SJ, Puhaindran ME, Lim AYT, Lim IJ, Bee WH. The Prevalence of Absence of the Palmaris Longus – A Study in a Chinese Population and a Review of the Literature. *Journal of Hand Surgery.* 2005; 30(5): 525–527.

64. Gonzalez MH, Whittum J, Kogan M, Weinzweig N. Variations of the Flexor Digitorum Superficialis Tendon of the Little Finger. *Journal of Hand Surgery.* 1997;22(2): 277–280.

65. Moore KL, Dalley AF, Agur AMR. *Clinically oriented anatomy.* 7th ed. Philadelphia: Wolters Kluwer/Lippincott Williams & Wilkins Health; 2014.

66. Dell PC, Sforzo CR. Ulnar Intrinsic Anatomy and Dysfunction. *Journal of Hand Therapy.* 2005;18(2): 198–207

67. Schünke M, Schulte E, Schumacher U. *THIEME Atlas of Anatomy: Head, Neck, and Neuroanatomy.* 2nd ed. New York: Thieme; 2016.

68. Riddoch G, Bristow WR, Cairns HWB, Carmichael EA, Critchley M, Greenfield J, et al. The Aids to the Examination of the Peripheral Nervous System (Memorandum No. 45). *Medical Research Council*; 1976.

69. Miller SF, Glasier CM, Griebel ML, Boop FA. Brachial plexopathy in infants after traumatic delivery: evaluation with MR imaging. *Radiology.* 1993;189(2): 481–484.

70. Bertelli JA, Ghizoni MF. Reconstruction of C5 and C6 brachial plexus avulsion injury by multiple nerve transfers: spinal accessory to suprascapular, ulnar fascicles to biceps branch, and triceps long or lateral head branch to axillary nerve. *The Journal of Hand Surgery.* 2004;29(1): 131–139.

71. Benjamin K. Part 1. Injuries To The Brachial Plexus. *Advances in Neonatal Care.* 2005;5(4): 181–189.

72. Talbot K. Motor neurone disease. *Postgraduate Medical Journal.* 2002;78(923): 513–519

73. Xu D, Guo X, Yang CY, Zhang LQ. Assessment of Hyperactive Reflexes in Patients with Spinal Cord Injury. *BioMed Research International.* 2015;2015: 1–8.

74. Bates B, Bickley LS, Hoekelman RA. *A guide to physical examination and history taking.* Philadelphia: Lippincott; 1995.

75. Krasin E. Review of the current methods in the diagnosis and treatment of scaphoid fractures. *Postgraduate Medical Journal.* 2001;77(906): 235–237

76. Hackney LA, Dodds SD. Assessment of scaphoid fracture healing. *Current Reviews in Musculoskeletal Medicine.* 2011;4(1): 16–22.

77. Delahunt E, McEntee BL, Kennelly C, Coughlan GF, Green BS. The adductor squeeze test: which is the optimal test position for eliciting maximum squeeze values and adductor muscle activity? *British Journal of Sports Medicine.* 2011;45(4): 345–345

78. Micheli LJ. *Encyclopedia of sports medicine.* London: SAGE; 2011.

79. Martin HD, Savage A, Braly BA, Palmer IJ, Beall DP, Kelly B. The Function of the Hip Capsular Ligaments: A Quantitative Report. *Arthroscopy: The Journal of Arthroscopic & Related Surgery.* 2008;24(2): 188–195.

80. McClung MR. Pathogenesis of osteoporotic hip fractures. *Clinical Cornerstone.* 2003;5: s22–s29.

81. Chatra P. Bursae around the knee joints. *Indian Journal of Radiology and Imaging.* 2012;22(1): 27.

82. Mcneil CJ, Raymer GH, Doherty TJ, Marsh GD, Rice CL. Geometry of a Weight-Bearing and Non-Weight-Bearing Bone in the Legs of Young, Old, and Very Old Men. *Calcified Tissue International.* 2009;85(1): 22–30.

83. D'Août K, Pataky T, Clercq DD, Aerts P. The effects of habitual footwear use: foot shape and function in native barefoot walkers. *Footwear Science.* 2009;1(2): 81–94.

84. Rigoard P. Atlas of anatomy of the peripheral nerves: The nerves of the limbs –. 1st ed. New York, NY: Springer; 2017.

85. Ertuglu LA, Karacan I, Yilmaz G, Türker KS. Standardization of the Jendrassik maneuver in Achilles tendon tap reflex. *Clinical Neurophysiology Practice.* 2018;3: 1–5.

86. Whiteley MS. *Understanding venous reflux: the cause of varicose veins and venous leg ulcers.* Guildford: Whiteley Publishing; 2013.

87. Novelline RA, Squire LF. *Squires fundamentals of radiology.* 6th ed. Cambridge, MA: Harvard University Press; 2004.

88. Seeram E. *Computed tomography: physical principles, clinical applications, and quality control.* 4th ed. St. Louis, MO: Elsevier; 2016.

89. Heit JJ, Iv M, Wintermark M. Imaging of Intracranial Hemorrhage. *Journal of Stroke.* 2017;19(1): 11–27.

90. Naidech AM. Intracranial Hemorrhage. *American Journal of Respiratory and Critical Care Medicine.* 2011;184(9): 998–1006.

91. 5 Westbrook C, Roth C, Talbot J. *MRI in practice.* 4th ed. Oxford: Wiley-Blackwell; 2014.